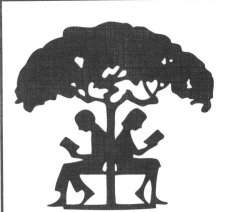

This book is a gift to the
Library by:
Genese Gibson

The Shadowmakers
A History of Radiologic Technology

The Shadowmakers
A History of Radiologic Technology

E.L. Harris

Edited by Paul T. Young
with Ceela McElveny and Barbara Pongracz-Bartha

A special project of the
American Society of Radiologic Technologists
commemorating its 75th Anniversary of service
to a noble profession.

Published by the American Society of Radiologic Technologists
15000 Central Avenue Southeast
Albuquerque, New Mexico 87123-3917

First edition printing, 2,000 copies, August 1995
IBSN# 1-886800-00-6

Printed in the United States of America

Author's Note

*I*t is always regrettable that the complexities of researching and writing a history, whether of an era, a business or profession, often cause the writer to overlook some individuals who played an integral part in that history. This is not done intentionally. The mass of information, archival material, printed documentation and individuals who shared their memories can overwhelm an unsuspecting author.

Even those few who can illuminate the beginnings of the American Society of Radiologic Technologists expressed during interviews their regret at "knowing I've forgotten to mention someone who was important to the association." If this is the case, apologies are in order. It is, however, the earnest wish of this author that those who might have been forgotten will be remembered as a result of this work.

In lieu of this, thanks are extended to the following for sharing their memories and their memorabilia: Frances Apple, Joan Baker, Bill Conklin, Sister Agnes Therese Duffy, Cindy Easterling, Edward Gunson, Laverne Gurley, Jack Heriard, Ruth Jaffke, Neta McKnight, Virginia Milligan, Royce Osborn, Theodore Ott, Juris Patrylak, Sister Marylu Stueber, Phyllis Thompson and Jane Van Valkenburg. Special thanks go to Genevieve Eilert, for the clarity of her memory, and to history buffs Jack and Angie Cullinan, for their years of careful documentation of the radiologic technologist's world.

For the ASRT staff, thanks go to Ward Keller, John Wade, Paul Young and Joan Parsons for their guidance; Ceela McElveny, Barbara Pongracz-Bartha and Nora Tuggle for their editorial contributions and photo research; and Katherine Ott, Marla Poteet and Robin Anderson for their proofreading and fact-checking. Thanks also must be extended to research contributor Pat Van Deusen, who has had an intimate relationship in the past few months with every dusty volume of *The X-Ray Technician* and *Radiologic Technology* ever printed. Last, but hardly least, I would like to thank graphic designer Kathleen Sparkes, who so elegantly pulled together the dangling manuscript components and wrapped them around a collection of hard-to-find photos and illustrations to make such a beautiful package.

The value of their work can only be equalled by the likes of Margaret Hoing, who so faithfully recorded the ASRT's history; by Alfred B. Greene, who documented the early years of the Registry; and to Professor Ed C. Jerman, who took the time to sit at an ancient Remington typewriter before his death and record his hopes, dreams and aspirations for a future generation.

E.L. Harris
Tijeras, New Mexico
1995

Dedication

This book chronicles the people whose research, leadership and personal sacrifice made an indelible mark on the profession of radiologic technology. The ASRT Board of Directors and staff dedicate this book to the members of the past 75 years and hope that it will serve as an inspiration to the members of the future.

In Memoriam

Paul T. Young, as ASRT marketing director, conceived the idea for *The Shadowmakers* and served as project manager and chief editor. Paul died on Jan. 27, 1995, before the book was finished. Those who worked closely with him committed themselves to completing the project so that *The Shadowmakers* would be published during this important year of the Roentgen Centennial and the 75th Anniversary of the American Society of Radiologic Technologists.

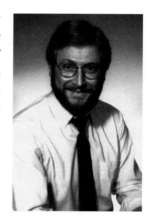

"Your profession and, indeed, your career are not limited to a single clinical setting or a single series of procedures. The radiologic sciences truly are among the most dynamic pursuits in all medicine. The issues are large and important, and your participation is vital."

— Paul T. Young
1952-1995

Preface

*H*istory is a living, breathing process, a constant convection fueling the future. It asks not recognition or even appreciation. And all too often it receives none, leaving those of the present deluded as to the context of their being. Are they majestic or minute? Once history passes by without recording, it can never be recaptured, much less understood.

This book, *The Shadowmakers*, is the first comprehensive history chronicling the struggles and accomplishments of a dedicated group of individuals whose contributions to the radiologic sciences and medical imaging have gone largely unrecognized. Since the discovery of x-rays by Wilhelm Conrad Roengten 100 years ago, the men and women of science and medicine have depended on associates to refine their theories and improve their practices.

These associates, early on referred to as "technicians," often sacrificed their health to advance medical science and patient care techniques. And their history has almost escaped us.

It is to these people whose legacy of sacrifice and dedication led to the modern profession of radiologic technology that we dedicate this book.

In 1995, the year of the Roentgen Centennial, the American Society of Radiologic Technologists celebrates its 75th Anniversary of service to a noble profession. We who have the privilege of leading this association feel the very deepest sense of pride in its long tradition. We hope this history provides all technologists in all the related disciplines this same feeling of pride.

Our practices today have not sprung full grown from some magical void. We are not mere accessories of convenience or extensions of some other profession's heritage. We have our own substantial lineage, our own traditions, heroes and martyrs. We have our own history and collective accomplishments. We have a most precious right to be proud of who we are and what we do. Please join us in celebrating *The Shadowmakers*.

Ward M. Keller
ASRT Chief Executive Officer

Table of Contents

Introduction

The period between the European Renaissance and the Age of Industrialization offered peculiar problems to the scientific community. By 1820 Mary Shelley's *Frankenstein* had created an image of the mad professor, working in solitary, manipulating electro-mechanical apparatus to produce the fantastic. Europeans, dosed with an appropriate amount of self-protective skepticism regarding science in general — and scientific discoveries in particular — tended toward stoic lassitude or outright ridicule.

The scientific community, always an insular body, was visited with its own healthy skepticism. Yet this was an age of discovery, and who discovered what was as important then as it is today. Credit for a discovery certainly didn't merit a financial windfall, but it did merit a credibility that in the 1890s was a commodity more important than money. Such was the world in which physicist Wilhelm Conrad Roentgen found himself.

Charles C Thomas Publisher

Roentgen's admission into German universities was delayed for three years after he was expelled from secondary school for failing to tell on a classmate prankster. In 1865 he finally was accepted to the Polytechnical School of Zurich in the mechanical engineering program. Roentgen's interest in physics was inspired by the experimental physicist August Kundt who taught at the university. Roentgen followed Kundt to the University of Strassburg in 1872, where he was named Privat Dozent, a mark of academic distinction that erased the teen-age scandal.

In 1888 the University of Würzburg offered Roentgen a position he couldn't refuse — professor of physics and director of the newly constructed Physical Institute. His appointment as head of a department at the university exemplified the respect and esteem Roentgen had earned.

Entombed within his basement laboratory at the University of Würzburg, this heavily-bearded, solitary German physicist fit Shelley's description of the mad scientist to a "T". Consider, for example, Roentgen's equipment: a lead battery, mechanical interrupter, Ruhmkorff spark inductor, discharge tube, vacuum pump, induction coil, Hittorf tube and a photographic plate. One wall of Roentgen's lab was described as a mass of wires, glass tubes and bottles in racks.

Some German biographers have described Roentgen as a classic savant — brilliant and driven in the area of his personal interests and completely unconcerned with practically all else. He was known for his persistence and critical honesty in making observations and measurements, for his thoroughness in approaching problems and for basing his experiments on firm theoretical foundation and logic.

Did Roentgen know what he was looking for? Perhaps. His experiments were based on those conducted by Sir William Crookes, German physicist Phillipp Lenard and perhaps even those of American experimenter Arthur Willis Goodspeed. Lenard and Goodspeed produced mysterious results, but they didn't quite comprehend what it was they had uncovered. On Nov. 8, 1895, Roentgen succeeded where they had failed.

He was repeating Lenard's experiments with cathode rays, expanding them to include a Hittorf-Crookes' tube. Roentgen was working with a tube covered with black cardboard when he saw fluorescent spots on a piece of barium platinocyanide paper on a table across the room. The fluorescence could only be caused by light, but the tube wasn't emitting light because it was shielded. Further tests at different distances and through various objects gave the same result. He named the discovery x-rays — "X" being the algebraic symbol for the unknown.

Later Roentgen told a friend, "I have discovered something interesting but I do not know whether or not my observations are correct." He spent the next seven weeks secluded in his laboratory, performing several experiments repeatedly to confirm the accuracy of his results. He even moved his bed into the laboratory to avoid the interruption of daily "trivialities" and in case he received sudden inspiration.

Roentgen persuaded his wife to be the subject for one of his experiments and exposed her hand to his new rays for 15 minutes. When Roentgen showed her the plate with skeletal image of her hand, she reportedly shuddered and said it created in her a dark foreboding — in her words: "a vague premonition of death."

On Saturday, Dec. 28, 1895, Roentgen submitted his first "provisional" communication, *Ueber eine neue Art von Strahlen* (On a New Kind of Rays), which was printed in the proceedings of the Würzburg Physico-Medical Society.

Because of the Christmas season, Roentgen presented his first oral discussion of his discovery on Jan. 23, 1896, and afterward produced a Roentgen ray image of the hand of anatomist Albert Rudolf von Kolliken. Interestingly enough, the linkage between the discovery of the x-ray and its application to the medical profession was immediate.

Although Roentgen refused to patent any part of his discovery, strongly rejecting all commercial offers, he did receive a number of distinctions, including the Hindenberg Iron Cross and the very first Nobel Prize in Physics in 1901. However, success was fleeting. Roentgen soon became embroiled in controversy when Phillipp Lenard claimed to be the true discoverer of the x-ray, and by the public's somewhat whimsical view of his invention's product.

Unlike other discoveries of the time, Roentgen's original experiments could be reproduced rather easily, as the necessary paraphernalia was readily available. Refinements were quick in coming, both in Europe and America. Hardly a month had passed after Roentgen's lecture when American Arthur Goodspeed suggested the term "radiography" be applied to cover the whole field of x-ray use.

But what about that use? How were physicians — that most secular group of scientists — expected to react to a discovery that could be duplicated easily by almost anyone with a basic understanding of electrical engineering? With grudging acceptance. Casual contempt. A need to contain and control. Considering that the international medical community had hardly risen above the use of leeches at the time, the x-ray's introduction created a dilemma.

Fortunately, there were those who immediately recognized a diagnostic tool offering unparalleled opportunities in advancing health care. While applications of the x-ray ranged from the sublime to the ridiculous, it was the medical community that eventually embraced, expanded and legitimized this tool into what it is today: a miracle of science.

But like all newly-found tools, those who developed its usage also tended to retard its growth because of their need to guard the purity of its intent. Protecting the x-ray from the unethical,

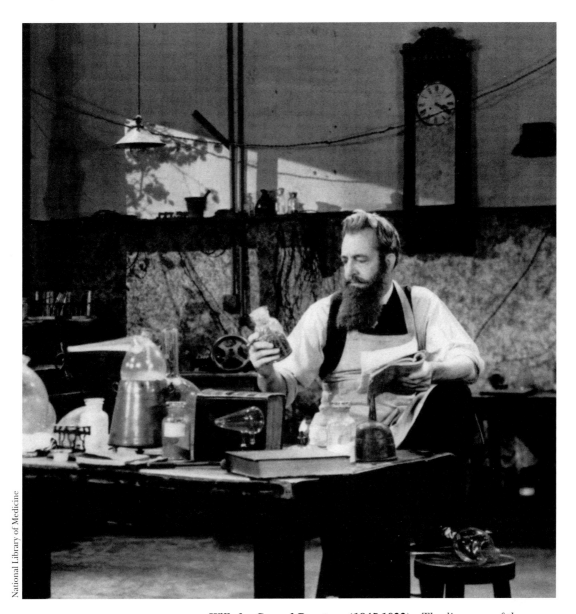

National Library of Medicine

Wilhelm Conrad Roentgen (1845-1922) - The discoverer of the x-ray.
He is shown above in his laboratory at the University of Würzburg.

the frivolous and the uneducated set the circuitous climb for those who would some day be called "technicians."

The relationship between doctor and technician would be a long struggle for understanding and professional credibility as the responsibility for performing diagnostic and therapeutic procedures shifted to medical specialists educated in anatomy, radiation safety and patient care — the radiologic technologists of today.

Chapter One

The Birth of a Science

When Wihelm Conrad Roentgen released news of his discovery, reactions were quick and predictable, even within the medical community. The *New York Medical Record* published an article characterizing Roentgen's discovery as "unimpressing." An 1896 editorial in the *London Electrical* belittled the discovery with the rationale that "very few people... would care to sit for a portrait which would show only the bones and the rings of the fingers."

Many lay individuals were horrified by the thought of rays that would reveal a person's interior. The British *Pall Mall Gazette* in March 1896 editorialized that the idea of seeing a human's bones was "a revolting indecency (on which) there is no need to dwell," and demanded from the government a "legislative restriction of the severest kind" for tungstate of calcium and its use in x-ray imaging.

Even Alan Archibald Campbell Swinton, the Scottish engineer who was possibly the first to produce an intentional roentgenogram after Roentgen, found x-ray images were not necessarily well received. In his autobiography, Swinton recalled that when he showed an x-ray plate of his own hand to the Prince of Wales in 1896 the Prince very ungraciously said, "How disgusting!"

Fortunately, not all people, lay or otherwise, felt this way. The American Medical Association (AMA), for example, began regularly commenting on the x-ray. In 1896 the *Journal of the American Medical Association* reported that x-rays were visible to insects (a rather odd observation) and, in a report from Vienna, that the electrical apparatus was so expensive — *$100 and upward* — that few surgeons could afford to use it in private practice.

While the AMA remained tastefully impartial to the x-ray and its applications, it nonetheless continued following the development. In 1897 the *Journal* reported that Dr. R.A. Fessenden of Western University developed an x-ray apparatus believed to be the "largest of its kind in the world: a coil weighing 175 pounds with 50 miles of wire and giving a spark 20 inches long. A photograph can be taken through the thickest part of the body in 15 minutes."

Practical applications of the x-ray also began appearing. In 1898 the *Journal* carried an article saying that "Ausset and Bedart report a case of tuberculosis peritonitis cured completely with 50 séances of 30 minutes each with the tube 20 centimeters from the skin." In another article it was reported that "Dr. A.H. Meisenbach of St. Louis located nails, staples, screws,

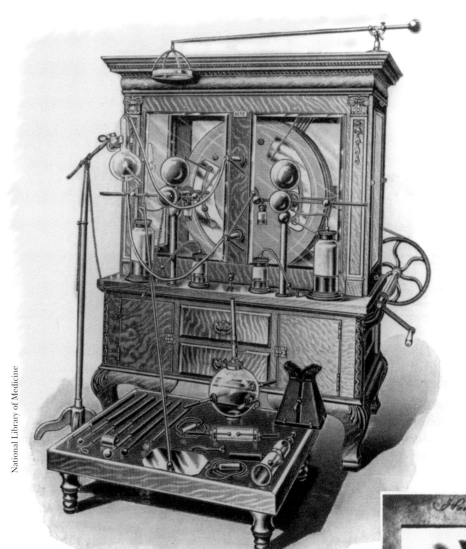

National Library of Medicine

Circa 1903 - *(left)*
an early model static machine
used for general x-ray work.
Note the handcrank on
the right.

Circa 1900 - *(lower left) x-ray*
laboratory of Wolfram Fuchs.

Circa 1895 - *(below right)*
the first x-ray taken of Anna
Bertha Ludwig Roentgen's
hand.

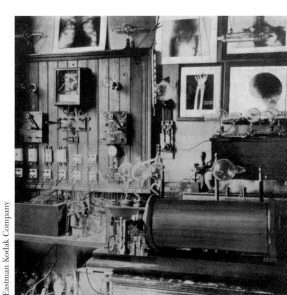

Eastman Kodak Company

Charles C Thomas Publisher

common nails, horseshoe nails, cartridges and a piece of chain in the stomach of a patient." Dr. Meisenbach claimed this was the first case on record in which x-rays were used to corroborate a diagnosis.

The good doctor used nearly five hours of exposure time, including fluoroscopic study, to obtain his results, but did not comment on his patient's diagnosis, nor on his rather peculiar diet. What was the world supposed to make of such reports?

> *Dr. A.H. Meisenbach of St. Louis located nails, staples, screws, common nails, horseshoe nails, cartridges and a piece of chain in the stomach of a patient.*

It was obvious that nothing could stop the development of the x-ray, but it was equally obvious why an air of cynicism existed. Whether used as a photographic novelty or a serious diagnostic tool, the x-ray found itself quickly immersed in the mainstream of human consciousness. Without the benefit of modern mass communication, progress of the x-ray's variety of applications was, as much as anything else, the print media's discovery of the century.

It was also a tool immediately recognized as a potential bonanza by the world's capitalists, both large and small. The x-ray was, after all, essentially a simple photographic process. Most radiographers were photographers or physicians who practiced photography as a hobby. Others were professors in university physics laboratories who were intrigued by x-rays as an addition to science. Others were amateur experimenters and inventors.

According to Wolfram Conrad Fuchs, who would eventually become a well-recognized diagnostician, "Many men attracted by the unknown... not well trained, but of an inquisitive mind or mechanical bent, procured the necessary apparatus to produce the new rays.

As many of the early experimenters had no medical and little scientific training, it was to these untrained investigators that medical men most often had to turn, for (radiography's) use demanded that it be obtained wherever possible."

Fuchs was speaking from experience. An electrician for the Cicero and Proviso Railroad, Fuchs was originally hired by two Chicago ophthalmologists to operate x-ray equipment. The venture proved to be so successful the Fuchs X-Ray Laboratory was soon established. It would herald the growth of an industry that many in the medical profession found ominous.

The "Roentgen studios" that appeared throughout Europe and America solicited physicians, mainly because physicians found the cost and operation of x-ray equipment difficult. Most of these studios' work was medical in nature, although they were known to provide radiographs of sculpture, jewelry, paintings and mummies, among other things, all of which foreshadowed modern industrial radiography.

One such studio purchased advertising space in the June 3, 1896, edition of the *Electrical Engineer*, stating: "Mr. M.F. Martin has opened an x-ray studio at 100 E. 26th Street in New York City, where pictures of interior human structure will be taken. The consultation hours are from 1:00 to 2:00 and from 5:00 to 6:00. A lady assistant is in attendance."

Another studio in Denver, operated by Colonel Charles F. Lacombe, offered a free x-ray service. The laboratory was besieged by people who were certain that their physicians were wrong in their diagnosis and wanted x-ray photographs to prove it. This prompted the Colonel to establish a prophetic rule that no patient would be x-rayed unless his physician was present.

The problem was that many in the American medical community thought that the results of x-rays were obvious, requiring no special interpretation. This would rapidly change. The European community, especially the Germans and the French, pressed forward with their own pragmatic development and refinement of the various types of equipment used to produce the x-ray.

The British, applying commonsense practicality to this new discovery, began to formalize the usage of the x-ray, perhaps understanding its real diagnostic potential for their highly structured approach to medical practice. And where the British led, the Americans were sure to follow, taking a good idea and expanding upon it. The first signs of American ingenuity appeared in the Spanish American War, where the military gave the x-ray a very practical application.

During the war with Spain, the United States Medical Corps used five static machines and 12 coils operated with primary batteries. Major J. Battersby of London, England, stated that after the battle of Omdurman, bullets were located in 20 patients when they could not be found by other means. Power for the x-ray machine was supplied from a small dynamo operated by a tandem bicycle. Other portable equipment was powered by "x-ray tricycles," airplane engines and horses.

Not to be outdone by the Army, the U.S. Navy followed suit. An article appearing in the September 1898 *Electrical World* stated: "When the Navy needed an x-ray outfit in a hurry, an Edison portable was installed in less than 48 hours from the time the order was received."

The portable was installed aboard the hospital ship "Solace," placed immediately in service and used in Santiago de Cuba during the Spanish War. It was heralded as the "very first floating x-ray equipment in the U.S. Navy."

While the United States military, especially in time of war, was capable of affording such "expensive" equipment, the only institutions other than the commercial Roentgen studios with the necessary funds were universities and major hospitals.

The first "clinical" radiograph believed taken in the United States is attributed to Edwin B. Frost, astronomy professor at Dartmouth College. Frost's physician brother asked him to radiograph the fractured forearm of a patient, which Frost did on Feb. 3, 1896, in a 20-minute exposure, successfully revealing the fracture.

Hospitals grudgingly provided limited resources, still considering x-rays a low priority. Massachusetts General Hospital in the fall of 1896 established what may have been the first x-ray department in the United States. In charge of this department was Walter J. Dodd, originally employed by the hospital as an apothecary. Because Dodd had shown a strong interest and skill in photography, he eventually became the hospital's official photographer. It was only natural that Dodd take over x-ray duties as well.

In 1899 Philadelphia General Hospital provided a special ground floor room, 12 by 15 feet, built of concrete. With 180 square feet of floor space, 3 square feet were separated for a photographic developing room, leaving a total space of 12 by 12 feet for the equipment and furnishings, which consisted of a Ruhmkorff coil, a small adjustable tube stand and Roentgen-ray tube.

With the x-ray treated as though it were a necessary evil of dubious value, it was a wonder that radiology ever emerged as a legitimate science. But the application of science, thanks to those who were unafraid of the rebuffs of peers, forged ahead in every major U.S. city. Despite the charlatans and the frivolous, there were those who foresaw the assets of the x-ray. Francis Henry Williams is often labeled as America's first radiologist. In April 1896 Williams enlisted patients at Boston City Hospital for his early studies, giving demonstrations at the Massachusetts Institute of Technology that showed the value of x-rays in diagnosing diseases of the thorax. He also encouraged physical experimentation before clinical trials, such as comparing the results of x-rays through clear water vs. bodily fluids. Based on his findings, Williams concluded that optimal medical diagnosis with x-rays depended on the differential opacity of air as opposed to water in organic tissue.

Despite Williams' successes, the established medical community continued to reject or accept new ideas based upon its existing accumulated body of knowledge — something severely lacking in radiology. With no textbooks and few precedents, early radiologists were forced to use "retrospectoscopy" to learn the x-ray manifestations of various disorders.

"Retrospectoscopy" involved the radiologist making plates, examining them and, more than likely, failing to make a sound diagnosis. The patient either was operated on or died and was examined at autopsy. The radiologist attended the operation or the autopsy and learned the true diagnosis. Then, in retrospect, the plates were re-examined and searched — often with embarrassment — for the clues that had been missed. The value of retrospectoscopy appeared in later examinations of other patients that revealed similar findings.

As radiographic techniques and equipment slowly improved, some x-ray operators acquired greater medical knowledge through osmosis. The lack — or complete void — of established educational standards and places where an aspiring x-ray practitioner could gain even slight knowledge further hampered professionalism.

Of even greater danger were those physicians, some of whom were failures in general practice and with little special knowledge, entering the field of x-ray. These men often possessed poor technical ability and were as dangerous in the practice of radiology as the nonmedical technician.

The problem was that despite the x-ray's rapid development, it was seen as a specialty. As individuals became more consumed with the lucrative aspects of x-ray, the wheels of deliberate science had not yet begun to grind, establishing true guidelines and practices. It would be many years in coming.

In 1910 Russell D. Carman of St. Louis, recognized as one of the most vigorous proponents of medical radiology as a specialty, complained that "the only valid criticism of the Roentgen ray is based on the fact that during its brief existence an abundance of poor work has been done with it by incompetent or inexperienced men, in many instances working with crude apparatus."

Carman added that when specialization was favored, "the pictorially excellent skiagraph of a hand or foot made by some enthusiastic amateur will no longer excite wonder, and the photographers, electricians and janitors who now make the so-called x-ray photographs in many hospitals will have their activities transferred to other fields where they will be less a menace to the public health."

The term "skiagraph" was a more elite name for an x-ray film, "skia" coming from the Greek, meaning shadow; thus the "shadowgraph."

Thirty years later J.T. Murphy would conclude that "a heritage still remains in the minds of many persons connected with medicine and hospitals; it is the idea that roentgenologists require no elaborate medical training. Many still feel that production of films of sufficient excellence is enough and that anyone can interpret them.

"This is much in evidence among surgeons and internists, men who would be the first to denounce the roentgenologist for removing

William Herbert Rollins

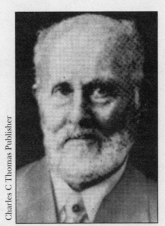

Charles C Thomas Publisher

The first major advocate for protection from radiation was William Herbert Rollins, a Boston dentist. In January 1898, Rollins suffered a severe x-ray burn that encouraged him to begin experimenting with guinea pigs. Determining that the adverse effects were a result of the x-rays, Rollins established three precautions: wearing radiopaque glasses; enclosing the x-ray tube in a leaded or other nonradiable housing; and irradiating only areas of interest by covering adjacent areas with radiopaque material.

Unfortunately, Rollins' suggestions were widely ignored, probably because he seldom attended meetings of the various societies dedicated to the study of x-rays. Even when finally awarded honorary membership in the American Roentgen Ray Society, the citation made no mention of Rollins' x-ray protection efforts.

Many radiologic specialists of the time scoffed at such findings. Ernest A. Codman, a noted surgeon-radiologist, charged Rollins with being overly dramatic and stated, "I believe that the comparatively small number of unfortunate cases which have been published circulated much farther than the immense number of fortunate cases, and have given the profession the idea that the process is a dangerous one to the patient."

an appendix… but who at the same time do not hesitate to diagnose a gastric ulcer from a set of roentgenograms made by a technician, even though in the present day system of medical training the roentgenologist is far better trained in surgery and medicine than the surgeon or the internist is in roentgenology."

Specialization, however, was destined to come and would be abetted by the nature of x-rays themselves. As more and more individuals — whether amateurs or serious professionals — experimented with the x-ray, it became increasingly obvious there were very real dangers associated with the process.

The many physicists, engineers, physicians and lay experimenters working with x-ray photography early on took no deliberate measures to protect themselves, their assistants or their patients from exposure to x-rays. There was no reason to expect any adverse physical effects from radiation. But accounts of serious damage eventually began to mount.

The *Electrical Review*, in its Aug. 12, 1896, issue mentioned the case of Herbert Hawks, who worked in Columbia University's x-ray lab as well as giving x-ray demonstrations at Bloomingdale Brothers. Hawks reported a drying of the skin, loss of hair and the eventual loss of skin on his hands. Doctors treated him for "parboiling." After Hawks improved, he went back to his x-rays, although he did protect himself, first with petroleum jelly, then a glove, then with tinfoil over his hand.

Other similar effects were noted in the first few years of x-ray use. Though not fully understood, it was recommended in 1921 that "all those who are employed in radiographic work or with radium have their blood examined periodically — every six months — as by doing so the disease could be recognized at a very early state, and probably be stopped."

Ironically, the medical literature of the early 1900s contained a number of cases in

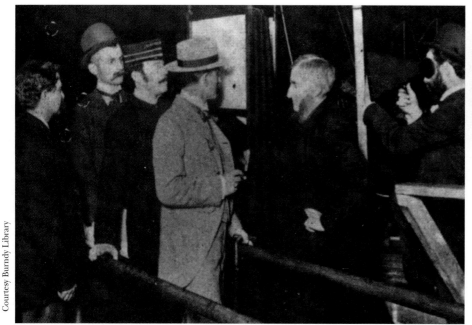

Courtesy Burndy Library

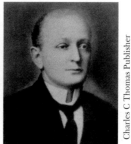

Charles C Thomas Publisher

1865-1904 – (above) Clarence Dally, Edison's assistant and the first x-ray martyr.

1896 – (left) People lined up to view their hands with Edison's fluoroscope at the National Electrical Exposition.

which patients suffering from skin cancers caused by x-ray burns were treated with additional x-rays in an effort to cure the cancers.

The most famous among this group was Clarence M. Dally, an assistant to Thomas Alva Edison, inventor of the fluoroscope. Actually, Edison's fluoroscope was an improvement of Italian Enrico Salvioni's 1896 invention, the "cryptoscope." After a demonstration of Edison's fluoroscope at his "Beneficent X-Ray Exhibit" at the 1896 Electrical Exposition in New York City, during which Dally was charged with adjusting the fluoroscope, the assistant began to suffer visibly from radiation. Edison immediately discontinued his experiments with x-rays, but it was too late for Dally, who died in 1904 — the first recorded radiation fatality.

The reasons for x-ray burns were ascribed to a number of things. Nikola Tesla, who developed the electric alternating current, was convinced it was not the rays, but the ozone generated by contact with the skin. Other theories included infectious material on the skin's surface, platinum particles from x-ray tubes, and the static current or charges induced in the tissue by the induction field surrounding the x-ray tube.

Whether or not the dangers of radiation had any impact on the number of people entering the profession or on the push for specialization is uncertain. What was apparent as the century came to a close was a wide divergence of opinion in and outside of the medical community. Without a firm consensus of opinion, it was evident there was a need to establish some sort of forum through which an exchange of information and ideas could circulate.

Enter Heber Robarts of St. Louis. In May 1897 Dr. Robarts launched a periodical he described as "a monthly journal devoted to practical x-ray work and allied arts and sciences." It was titled *The American X-Ray Journal.* Robarts later said, "In starting the journal I did not consult anyone about the propriety or wisdom of my course. If I had it would have been swallowed up by the historic monster of disapproval." At that time there seemed to come a famine or spell over the Roentgen world. The lay press had already ceased to print sensational matter about the x-rays and medical journals were not certain that the profession could read skiagraphs.

Robarts' editorial in the first issue offered reasons why he thought physicians were not readily adopting the "new science" even though the public was eager for its use. He reviewed the application of the new rays in some surgical situations, stressing the "ease and certainty of diagnosticating which has advanced more in the past 12 months than any previous hundred years" and promised that the *X-Ray Journal* would provide only truthful results concerning x-ray work from around the globe.

He also wrote that the new field of x-ray had to be associated with "practical and useful adjuncts," the most important being medical jurisprudence, the therapy of electro-medical science, preventive medicine, hygiene, dentistry and collateral branches. Robarts also asserted that no advertisements suggesting "quackery, deception or fraud" would appear, and that as editor, he would see that the journal's content would be ethical without being arrogant, biased or defiant.

Robarts obviously recognized the establishment with which he competed. The prestigious *Journal of the American Medical Association* continued to receive the lion's share of original research papers, relegating Robarts to reprints on radiology from other sources. But Robarts had found a niche, gained credibility within his peer group, and was sufficiently inspired to take the next step — the founding of a society dedicated to the development of x-ray science.

In 1900 the Roentgen Society was founded with Robarts as its president. Much discussion centered on whether this new organization should seek the blessings of the AMA and whether its membership should be limited to physicians in good standing with the AMA or open to nonphysicians and physicians on the outs with the AMA, such as electrotherapists.

The decision was made to proceed without the AMA, as it was felt that the society needed the physicists' and electrotherapists' support more.

Thus the membership was open to physicians and radiographers, as well as inventors, technical electricians, chemists and others. Though Robarts' *X-Ray Journal* requested that "no quacks or fakes of whatsoever sort need apply," this was never clearly defined. In fact, any of the *X-Ray Journal's* subscribers without credentials could gain membership in the Roentgen Society if they were members of a

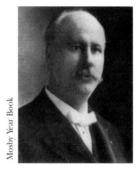

*1852-1922 – (left)
Heber Robarts, founder
of* The American
X-Ray Journal.
*Shown below is the
cover of the first issue.*

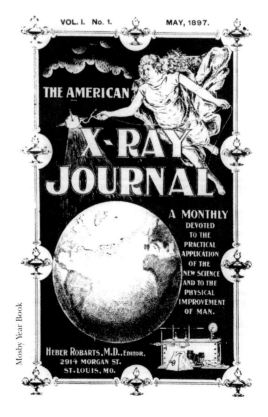

medical or other scientific society and paid $5 dues.

The first meeting of the Roentgen Society was in New York City on Dec. 13-14, 1900. It brought together a 150-member audience that listened to 25 papers and viewed extensive exhibits of x-ray appliances that displayed "the tremendous strides to have been taken in the short life of the industry."

However, this and the 1901 session revealed some of the problems of radiology at the time. Robarts seemed to embody the plight of the roentgenologist, who was "engulfed with electrotherapists to the left of him, jealous x-ray neophytes to the right of him, and up-start manufacturers in front of him." Apparently disgruntled by the large number of nonmedical members in the society, Robarts declined re-election and later resigned his membership.

The impetus begun by Robarts, however, could not be denied. By the time of the third annual society meeting in Chicago in 1902, those physicians aligned with the AMA had gained control over the organization. It was renamed the American Roentgen Ray Society (ARRS). The radiologist had at last gained a respectable forum for recognition.

One of the primary thrusts of the ARRS was its insistence from its beginning that radiology be integrated into the profession of medicine, that its practice be the practice of medicine, its practitioners be broadly trained in general medicine, and the radiologist preserve his own freedom and autonomy as a practicing physician.

By 1905 the ARRS had purged itself of "undesirable elements." Many Western members resigned or were dropped for nonpayment of dues. The ARRS effectively became an honor society for the elite, controlled by East Coast physicians.

But the Midwestern colleges were producing a number of graduates who were gaining

national stature. They had fewer ties with Europe and less inherent respect for established East Coast authority. The door to respectability for these individuals would not long remain closed.

The practice of medicine was certainly not limited to the East Coast elite, nor to big city hospitals. The U.S. population was expanding rapidly westward, carrying with it a host of general practitioners and surgeons whose time was best spent worrying about the health of their patients rather than their own standing in a society. Surprisingly enough, the adjuncts of x-ray equipment were developing faster than the societies that had hoped to control them, and the general practitioners in rural Iowa and Colorado found themselves faced with an array of x-ray equipment that was relatively inexpensive and simple to operate.

Indeed, manufacturers worldwide had jumped on Roentgen's bandwagon by that point. The first advertisement for x-ray equipment appeared in the classified section of *Neue Freie Presse*, Vienna, the same day Roentgen delivered his oral presentation. By May of that same year, the British firm B.J. Edwards & Company began marketing a short-lived "cathodal plate," which was a photographic plate with fluorescent salts incorporated into the emulsion.

Americans were not far behind. American manufacturing was in bloom. Hardly six months after Roentgen's announcement of his discovery, Philadelphia's Willyoung Company began marketing equipment, including a Roentgen machine consisting of a coil with a motor-operated rotary interruptor. It used a Bowdoin focusing x-ray tube, named after two physics professors at Bowdoin College. William Scheidel & Company of Chicago produced the first x-ray coil sold to a physician, Dr. Benjamin Hamilton of Shawnee, Oklahoma. In the August 1898 edition of *Electrical World*, General Electric advertised its production of a complete line of x-ray apparatus — the first company to produce equipment specific to the growing x-ray industry.

Morris E. Leeds & Company of Philadelphia introduced the Leeds 1901 Type Portable Induction Coil, which was easily transported in two cases. It was this type of portable coil that was purchased by the St. Louis X-Ray Laboratory, Montreal General Hospital, and St. Joseph's Hospital in Pennsylvania.

An article by William James Morton in February 1896 claimed that Roentgen rays were produced in open air between the discharge rods of a static machine. So static machines suddenly became a part of the x-ray industry, even though the most well known of these, the Patee Static Machine, had found primary use in demonstrating the effectiveness of lightning rods.

Leo Carl Kotraschek, in his *Outline of the X-ray Industry*, wrote: "The development of electrical and mechanical improvements in x-ray apparatus was a slow process. I feel that the radiologic fraternity owes a debt of gratitude to the host of x-ray salesmen, the detail men and service men, as they were during all that formative period the disseminators of news, techniques and development, being at the same time good listeners."

As improvements in x-ray equipment continued, other materials vital to the science were not as rapid in coming. Tubes of all types were in short supply and after early 1896 could only be found on back order. As a result, several light bulb companies began to include x-ray tubes in their lines.

Photographic plates were another matter altogether. The first glass plate specifically designed for x-ray imaging was introduced in 1896 by John Carbutt of Philadelphia. The 14-by-17-inch plate was quite expensive — $1 — half of what a modern film of the same size costs today.

Developing and fixing took as long as four hours. Even worse than the cost and time was the potential hazard to the doctor or operator — not to mention the patient — when the glass plates broke, as they all too often did from the weight of the patient. Many operators were cut by glass shards.

Yet an even greater hazard was the use of glass plates for dental x-rays, which required a glass cutter, a ruler and a sensitive plate. The plates were cut into bits about the size of present-day dental film. According to F.S. O'Hara, author of an article in a 1932 issue of *Radiography and Clinical Photography*, "by the time a half-dozen pictures of the teeth were made, the patient was bleeding from the gums like a baited bull in the bull ring."

All of this would, of course, change — and change rapidly. The development of the x-ray, whether as a diagnostic tool or a dangerous toy, never suffered from inertia. What it did suffer from was a spontaneous and unbridled growth that far outpaced the medical community's ability to apply professional standards to its use. By 1905 the radiologist was trapped in a never-never land; his services were in great demand but his integrity and methodology were questioned by others within the profession.

This paranoia, whether fueled by legitimate concern or common envy, drove men like Heber Robarts out of the profession and into seclusion. But the even larger question yet to be asked was: If it took such effort for the radiologist to gain credibility, what could x-ray technicians expect to encounter when the harsh light of medical scrutiny fell upon their work?

Putting the X-Ray to Work

When Wilhelm Conrad Roentgen produced the first human radiograph on Nov. 8, 1895, Charity Hospital in New Orleans, La., already was 159 years old. The story of this prestigious institution's struggle to acquire and adapt Roentgen's new technology offers insight into the evolution of radiology departments at hospitals throughout the United States.

The discovery of the x-ray was enthusiastically embraced by the New Orleans medical community. An editorial in the March 1896 issue of the *New Orleans Medical and Surgical Journal* optimistically predicted, "Away with your stethoscope, plessi-meter, sphymograph, opthalmoscope, laryngoscope and cystoscope! Away with your powder and pills, your knives and batteries! Bring forth your camera and your x-ray — there you have diagnosis, prognosis and treatment!"

Recognizing the technology's potential, Charity Hospital acted quickly to establish its own radiology department and installed a Roentgen ray apparatus before the end of 1896. Initially, the technology was used primarily to locate foreign objects and detect fractures. Often, the crude apparatus was incapable of performing even those rudimentary tasks. In August 1898, Dr. S.P. DeLaup described an attempt to use the Charity x-ray unit to locate a bullet in a patient. In a case presentation before the Louisiana Medical Society, DeLaup stated that "x-ray was decided upon, but the machine was out of order and a week was lost waiting." When the "skiagraph" finally was taken, another week was lost waiting for it to be developed, "which proved a failure." The bullet eventually was located through physical examination.

The dilemma of timely plate development was

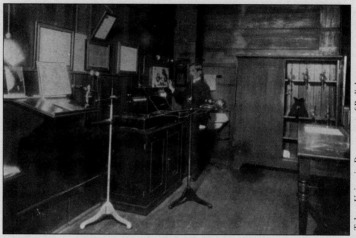

Circa 1900 — *The Charity Hospital x-ray department. An unidentified man is operating a generator connected to an x-ray tube attached to a floor stand. Patients stood in front of the x-ray tube while the roentgenologist viewed their anatomy through a hand-held Edison fluoroscope.*

Tulane University Department of Radiology

solved in 1899 when Charity Hospital built its first x-ray darkroom. Improvements in the department's equipment continued in 1902 with the installation of a 16-inch Sparks X-Ray Coil and Finsen's Ultraviolet Apparatus. In 1905 the x-ray room was renovated and "every instrument of precision used in radiography" was procured — a testament to the hospital's confidence in the new technology. Also in 1905, the radiology department was placed under the direction of Dr. Amedee Granger, a 1901 graduate of the Tulane University School of Medicine. Granger's small department produced an average of 15 diagnostic radiographs per month during 1905; by 1906, the figure had grown to more than 50 per month.

Under Granger's supervision, the radiology department gained a recognized place in the New Orleans medical community. Charity Hospital's 1908 annual report noted, "The increasing importance of the x-ray work to both the surgical and medical services makes it quite indispensable as there are many evidences that the work has bestowed incalculable advantages upon a certain class of patients.... As we now have one of the most complete x-ray laboratories, we feel sure that the work in this department will continue to increase."

The hospital's radiology department was expanded again in 1914 when it was partitioned into two rooms, one for skiagraph work and the other for fluoroscopy. A 2-kilowatt Schiedel-Western x-ray machine, fluoroscopic table, x-ray film illuminator and Granger x-ray frame — designed by Dr. Granger to assist in patient positioning during exposures — were added to the department.

On July 1, 1915, James B. Harney, M.D., was appointed resident roentgenologist at Charity Hospital. In his first six months as department director, 2,516 exposures were made on 1,720 x-ray exams of 1,686 patients. By 1919, the number of patients examined radiographically had increased to 8,799, and by 1920 the number had grown to 12,071. A Klinoscope and Coolidge tube were installed in 1919.

Harney resigned from Charity Hospital in 1920, and Granger again was appointed director of the department. During the next several years, many visiting roentgenologists from around the country spent one or two years at Charity Hospital under the training of Granger. These early roentgenologists not only interpreted the radiographic images, but also performed most of the examinations. Nurses and trained assistants helped with the patients and manned the darkroom to develop the films.

In 1921 Charity Hospital renovated its radiology department again. It had a complete filing system installed in a fire-proof vault, a 119-square-foot darkroom with tanks that could accommodate 75 films, three diagnostic x-ray units and one unit for x-ray treatments. A mobile x-ray unit was added in 1922.

In 1924 Martin T. Van Studdiford, M.D., joined the staff as director of radiation therapy. Prior to his appointment, Charity physicians purchased their own radium for use on their patients. Van Studdiford tightened control over radium use, but some errors still occurred. On April 21, 1931, 50 milligrams of radium valued at $3,500 were lost. The *New Orleans Morning Tribune* on May 19 reported that the radium, being used to treat a female patient, accidentally was placed into a bedside pan and subsequently was poured down the drain. The radium was traced through the sewers to a point near the river. This incident was the second time in two years that radium had been lost. To alleviate the problem, the hospital installed a Westinghouse deep therapy unit in July 1931.

The evolution of Charity Hospital's radiology department was typical of the era, dominated by struggles to acquire increasingly sophisticated technology and a need for acceptance by the mainstream medical community. Today, Charity Hospital is known as the Medical Center of Louisiana at New Orleans. Its radiology department continues serving the people of New Orleans from its fifth structure, opened in 1940.

— *Jack B. Heriard, R.T.(R)*
Tulane University Medical Center
Hospital and Clinic
New Orleans, La.

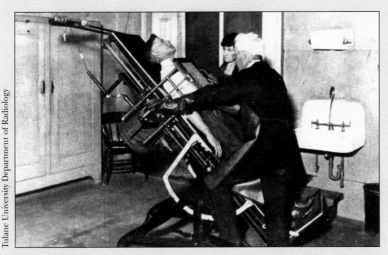

Tulane University Department of Radiology

Circa 1919 — *A Schiedel-Western fluoroscopic machine in use at Charity Hospital.*

Chapter Two

Enter the Specialists

In 1910 the American Roentgen Ray Society surveyed its members to define exactly who radiologists were and what training they had received. The great majority of respondents had acquired their medical degrees between 1896 and 1903, leaving the ARRS to conclude that "the specialty in 1910 was staffed with mostly younger men, many still pursuing studies when Roentgen's discovery was announced."

Among those receiving degrees between 1900 and 1903, a considerable number had begun working with x-rays in 1896 and 1897 as physicists, engineers, electricians, photographers or in other technical capacities. The ARRS found that these individuals — including Mihran Kassabian, Eugene Caldwell and Walter Dodd, later considered leaders in the field of radiology — had returned to school and earned their medical degrees specifically to qualify as radiologists.

The survey also indicated that only 20 percent of ARRS members were limiting their practice to radiology. The remainder were almost equally divided between general practice and some other specialty. But almost all respondents agreed the demand for x-ray services was increasing.

There still was no consensus of opinion,

however, within the ARRS regarding how best to establish the professional respect they believed radiology deserved. Divisions inside ARRS were often contentious. Two years prior to the ARRS survey, one member noted that "medical radiography was a piebald proceeding... which fit no one. The attendant wires and sparks suggested an electrician's work, surely... but there were the plates, darkroom and chemicals, considered usually the accessories of the photographer. Neither of these artisans, on the other hand, could be expected to intrude themselves so far into the realms of medicine as to offer a diagnostic verdict."

Interestingly, the above 1908 quote and the 1910 ARRS survey are attributed to the same man, one Dr. Percy Brown of Boston — also known as the hagiographer (one who writes about saints) of American radiation martyrs.

One of Brown's colleagues in ARRS, Dr. Russell D. Carman, countered that proper x- ray use "demands an intimate knowledge of a highly complex apparatus, practical acquaintance with the essentials of a good radiogram, ability to interpret bodies, familiarity with the therapeutic use of the rays, and appreciation of the dangers which may attend their careless or unskilled application."

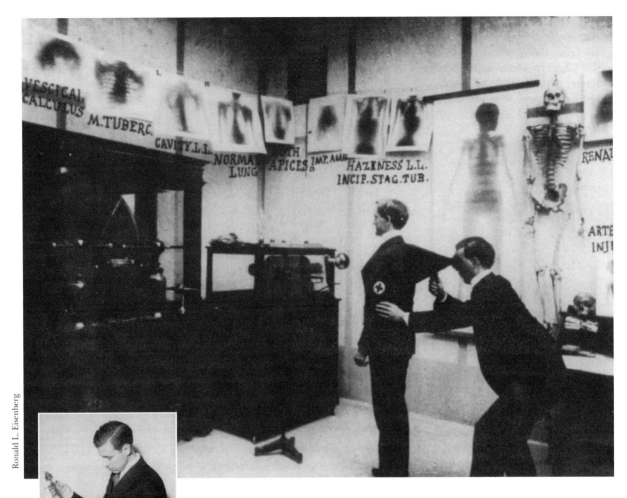

Ronald L. Eisenberg

General Electric Company

Circa 1901 - *(top) Kassabian's x-ray laboratory.*

Circa 1931 - *(left) General Electric 440 kVp tube.*

Circa 1901 - *(below) An early ARRS meeting held in Buffalo, N.Y.*

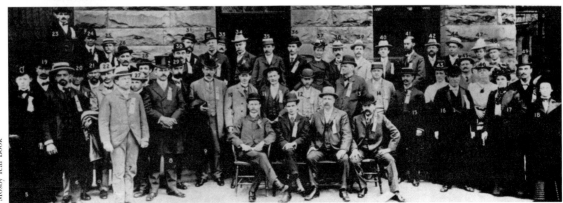

Mosby Year Book

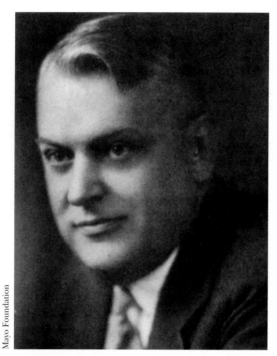

Mayo Foundation

1875-1926 - *Russell D. Carman*

Carman conceded, however: "There are in the United States today barely a dozen roentgenologists who are capable of performing really expert service."

Was Carman trying to shame his fellow ARRS members into a higher level of consciousness? The need was certainly apparent when considering the opinions of medical establishments outside the few ARRS Eastern edifices. A letter written as late as 1911 from Peter Bent Brigham Hospital stated that the hospital saw no need for the services of a roentgenologist, specifying, "In regard to a roentgenologist, we have put down no salary figure. The Department will probably involve the employment of one or more technical assistants, not graduates in medicine, with the probable supervision of a resident or visiting graduate in medicine."

One reason for the generally low opinion of radiologists among other specialists was that during this time radiologists were not willing to delegate the operation of their x-ray machines. Thus, they were perceived as

ranking somewhat lower than physicians — more like technicians. And if the radiologists had to bear such abuse, it was apparent the technicians who followed would eventually inherit these attitudes.

Even Brown of Boston observed the logical, natural progression from a distinct "premedical" stage, during which radiology or any other newly emerging discipline was in lay hands. Teaching radiology at the college level was slow in developing partly because of the required familiarity with electrophysics and the technical experience of manipulating fairly intricate apparatus. The earliest radiology books were nothing more than popular "how-to" guides outlining the fundamental principles of x-ray. These books combined a wealth of technical illustrations with examples of the few images available in the first several months following Roentgen's announcement of his discovery.

The first truly comprehensive American textbook was *The Roentgen Rays in Medicine and Surgery,* published by Francis Williams in 1901. This and subsequent books dealt with the wide spectrum of clinical applications of x-rays and were written to serve as overall reference sources for all physicians actively engaged in x-ray work.

Most of these books discussed the nature and properties of x-rays, then described various types of x-ray equipment and practical hints for positioning the patient, as well as the classic images showing the then-known variety of disorders of the bones, joints, heart and lungs and abdomen. After 1910 textbooks began to appear that were devoted to specific areas of diagnostic imaging and designed for specific use by radiologists, either those in training or in full-time practice.

Even so, as late as 1930 few American universities offered a diploma for the completion of postgraduate work in radiology. A number of teaching centers offered one- or two-year fellowships in radiology, but the courses lacked uniformity and proper scope. They were targeted to physicians who did not possess essential preliminary grounding in the basic principles of physics and radiologic technique.

Many postgraduate courses focused on certain specialties that relied heavily on radiology — gastroenterology and urology, for example. A majority of physicians seeking special instruction in radiology were content with a brief course of instruction, which could be obtained in an x-ray department of "dubious distinction" or simply by spending a few weeks looking over the shoulder of a practicing radiologist.

In 1933 radiologist and educator James T. Case described the relation of early radiologists to one another as "much like that of a group of widely separated research workers devoted to problems of common interest." Young physicians committed to radiology learned at the elbows of the pioneers, some going so far as to visit the various radiologic centers of Europe.

One can easily understand the frustration of men such as Case who decried "the vicious tendency on the part of incompetent or dishonest laymen, and even by unscrupulous physicians, to commercialize radiology (which) is a natural danger of too rapid expansion of the specialty of radiology and a consequent faulty and insufficient training of physicians entering it."

But such complaints barely whispered against the roar. Rapid expansion was the pace of the day, and radiologists trying to keep up would feel pressure like never before.

The unstoppable force came in the form of an ordinary human being, traveling from town to town, offering for sale the latest advancements in x-ray equipment. The traveling salesman would make x-ray imaging more accessible, more affordable and perhaps most importantly, more necessary.

After all, here was the greatest invention of the new 20th century, ready and waiting to serve an eager public. One can easily imagine the sales spiel, and the doctor who suddenly realized his practice would suffer from the lack of such equipment. Traveling ambassadors from the Victor X-Ray Company, from Picker and from another dozen companies ensured that no general practitioner or surgeon should remain ignorant of the benefits of x-ray. To prove it, the salesman brought with him the basic knowledge to demonstrate the equipment and even throw in a bit of diagnostic wizardry.

This was America in its heyday. Telephone and electrical power lines snaked into all corners of the country. Automobiles by the thousands rolled off smoking assembly lines. Black gold gushed like giant fountains from the ground in Texas and California. American technology was picking up speed like a runaway train, and the x-ray rode the leading edge.

The dilemma for the doctor — whether in small town middle America or metropolitan New York — remained the same. More and more of his time was eaten up by the mechanics of the x-ray, leaving less time for patient contact and treatment. Embracing finally the ideas of many within the ARRS, physicians such as general practitioners, surgeons and even radiologists realized that to make the most effective use of their x-ray equipment,

> **'**
> *The vicious tendency on the part of incompetent or dishonest laymen, and even by unscrupulous physicians, to commercialize radiology (which) is a natural danger of too rapid expansion of the specialty of radiology and a consequent faulty and insufficient training of physicians entering it.*
> **,**

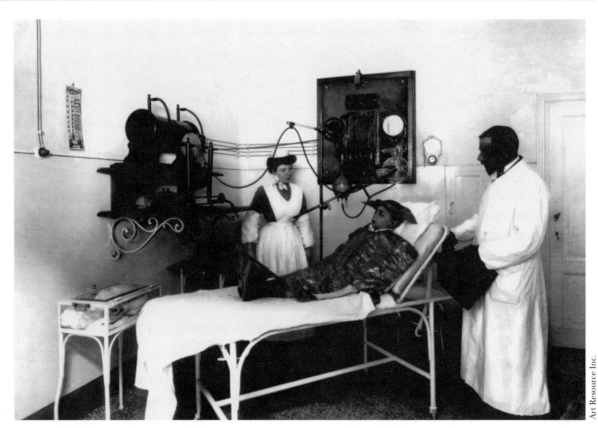

Art Resource Inc.

Circa 1900 - *An early x-ray therapy session.*

someone else had to handle the time-consuming tasks of taking and developing the x-ray films.

The task most often fell to the physicians' office assistants. Across the country physicians recruited their secretaries and receptionists to crank the handle of the static machine, pose as subjects and rock the developer pan. The pioneer technicians had a heavy load to bear. The vast majority were women, and they were expected not only to operate the x-ray equipment, but also to perform routine maintenance and repair minor breakdowns. These assistants usually had no knowledge of human anatomy or illness; they merely operated the equipment. Physicians lucky enough to employ nurses quickly put them to work as x-ray technicians, for they at least had medical training.

The role of the technician as an x-ray oper-

ator or "manipulator" might best be compared to that of the military conscript — enlisted without warning, and often without choice if they cared to continue receiving a paycheck — suddenly thrust into a duty that was foreign and, even for the trained nurse, somewhat frightening.

By 1914 another factor came into play, forcing the role of technician squarely on to the shoulders of women. World War I had begun, and many of the men who would have ordinarily assumed this role went off to war.

The war also created an unprecedented demand for x-ray technicians to staff military hospitals — the first of many personnel shortages to affect the profession.

Fortunately, the task of taking and developing x-rays had become easier and safer. By 1913 George Eastman had developed a special film with an x-ray sensitive emulsion coating, and refined it further in 1918 with a two-sided high speed emulsion coating. Technicians then were freed from the hazards of the old emulsion-coated glass plates — at least in more modern laboratories.

As late as 1909 the x-ray table was nothing more than a wooden bench. The x-ray tube, which still had no shielding around it, was clamped to a simple wooden tripod and energized by a static machine driven by a hand crank or direct current motor. The output of the static machine was approximately 100 kVp at 0.5 to 1.0 mA. Exposures of the hand required several minutes; 20 minutes or longer for a hip.

The darkrooms were sometimes set up by separating part of the x-ray room with a curtain. Consequently, developed plates often fogged. Many of the newly recruited technicians improvised, using homemade developing tanks that often were set up in a convenient bathroom — although running water and drying the film weren't considered absolutely necessary.

Learning at the hands of their mentors, technicians positioned patients by first observing, then doing, then adapting. Once the radiologist was convinced the technician was reasonably competent in the mechanical aspects, they were often left to experiment on their own.

Discovering what did and didn't work became known as the "hunch method" — taking x-rays by what felt right, not by any specific amount of exposure time. Technicians had to guess at patient density, calibration of the x-ray generator and the speed and quality of x-ray films. Apparatus was crude; timers did not exist on early equipment and voltage and current could not be accurately measured or controlled. The results often were overexposed film, and the technician would all too often try to compensate by underdeveloping the plates. This, of course, produced a very poor quality image.

Because of their status, technicians often found themselves performing their duties in a professional vacuum. With little or no opportunity to compare notes with others in their profession, they were left to prospect for whatever reading material was available, hoping to achieve at least a satisfactory performance for their radiologist.

With no standard rules, however, technicians found it difficult to explain their successes and could not formulate a technique that others could follow. With no standardized safety programs in place, technicians began to take their own precautions. Lead-impregnated aprons, jackets, gloves and x-ray-proof goggles came into popular use. While these steps helped alleviate some of the problems, the demands of World War I overwhelmed existing x-ray facilities and operators, resulting in a large number of poorly trained technicians who didn't fully realize the dangers. They held difficult patients for each other, used their own hands to test fluoroscopic tubes and stepped in front of the beam to prove to frightened patients that the procedure would not hurt.

After the war, there were calls for change. Charles L. Leonard, in his paper *Protection of Roentgenologists*, encouraged the medical community to seek out technical knowledge and clinical experience in operating x-ray equipment. He also urged the use of protective shields around the tube to cut off scatter radiation, and decried the carelessness of operators who left tubes unshielded but moved behind lead screens themselves, indicating that unnecessary radiation was being produced in the room. Finally, Leonard criticized equipment manufacturers for their lack of safety devices.

Otherwise, the plight of the technician went largely ignored and unnoticed. Their radiologist mentors were concerned with other matters

— dissatisfaction with the ARRS was brewing.

Prior to 1915 two of the largest specialty societies outside the ARRS were the Chicago Roentgen Society and the New York Roentgen Society. The latter group adopted an eight-point Code of Ethics recommending that x-ray examinations be performed only on a doctor's referral or personal knowledge of the patient. It also approved guidelines for advertising radiographic services and policies for releasing radiographs to patients.

Despite their progressive ways and separate identities from ARRS, these two associations excluded many practicing radiologists. In 1915 that changed.

St. Louis physician Edwin C. Ernst met with Fred Summa O'Hara, Heber Robarts' former secretary, to form a new open-door association of Roentgen ray specialists. Among the architects was George W. Brady of Chicago, the head of an x-ray equipment manufacturing company. Brady was encouraged to send letters to radiologists, hospitals and technicians in Missouri, Illinois and Iowa to see how they felt about such an organization.

The response was positive except for a few who eschewed the presence of lay workers. The first organizational meeting was Dec. 15-16, 1915, in Chicago, with about 30 charter members present out of a total of 62. O'Hara was named president of the group, which was christened the Western Roentgen Society (WRS). It staged its first scientific session in St. Louis the following year.

The ARRS *American Journal of Roentgenology* failed to mention this scientific meeting or even note the formation of the WRS. But neither the Midwestern radiologists, nor those throughout the rest of the country ignored by the ARRS, would be denied. Within four years of its appearance as a regional society, the Western Roentgen Society grew into a national organization, with 472 members in 38 states. Such overwhelming success prompted

a name change to the Radiological Society of North America (RSNA) in 1920.

It was later stated that the motive for founding the RSNA was "the firm belief held by its founders that there should be a place in organized radiology for young men, who should be encouraged to develop within the organization. The founders and older members of the RSNA have been proud of the fact that no member, regardless of his obscurity or the modesty of his attainment, has ever been denied the right to raise his voice in either the scientific or the executive sessions of the society."

In many ways, the success of the RSNA heralded an end to the East Coast dynasty and its exclusionary policies. But a wider acceptance of radiologists also brought the pressures of specialization back into focus. The need to separate the professional from the lay individual became apparent to the AMA, and the next call for credibility came from the West Coast.

In a 1923 meeting of the AMA in San Francisco, Dr. Albert Soiland of Los Angeles decried the lack of recognition received by radiology in American medical circles. Soiland wanted to create an organization committed to exclusivity, and so proposed the creation of the American College of Radiology (ACR). It was accepted.

As proposed by Soiland, the ACR would have a limited membership of 100 outstanding Fellows "who have distinguished themselves in the science of radiology... (having graduated from) a reputable institution of medicine and surgery and having devoted at least ten years to radiology." Soiland's ultimate goal was to force recognition of radiology as a legitimate and essential part of the medical community, and of radiologists as highly skilled professionals, "to make radiology a respected and useful branch of general medicine."

Although the AMA eventually would ac-

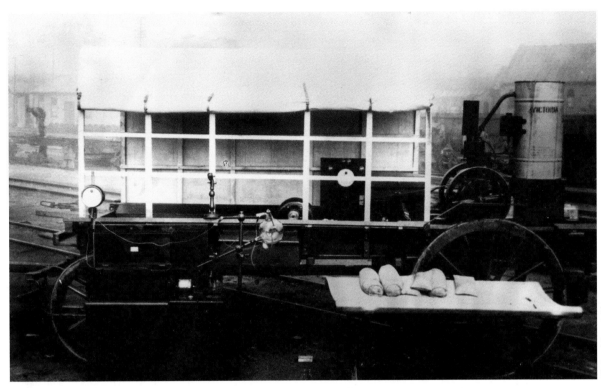

National Atomic Museum

Circa 1915 - *A World War I x-ray setup.*

cede to these wishes, the road to success was rough. As far back as the 1912 meeting of the AMA in Atlantic City, N.J., radiologists complained that "the space for Roentgen plates was confined to an out-of-the-way gallery with absolutely no conveniences provided for those who might desire to exhibit." At the 1913 meeting, the radiological exhibit was "placed upon the top floor of the scientific building and it required a maximum of enthusiasm to climb the flight of stairs."

In 1923 when Soiland pushed for creation of the ACR, he also urged the addition of a new official Section of Radiology to the AMA's existing 15 sections. Soiland pointed out that 1,000 members of the AMA were engaged full-time or part-time in the practice of radiology, and he warned that various state bodies were attempting to legalize and license the practice of radiology by laymen.

Although the AMA recommended that each section include in its program at least one paper pertaining to some other specialty, such as radiology, it refused to create a new section until 1925, when it finally bowed to the pressure of numerous members. Although a number of medical biographers have dealt with this period of time regarding the advancement of radiology, none specifically mentions why such pressure was so important and all-consuming. But Soiland may have given the best clue.

Legislation legalizing the practice of radiology — opening it to laymen — would have been one strong reason. Further legitimization of the Roentgen studios posed a direct threat to all radiologists and the credibility of their profession. However, what really drove the change was technology. Specifically, the Keletron Techron generator, the forerunner of all the anatomically programmed x-ray units to come. The Keleket X-Ray Corporation developed a "penetration per part" technique that would standardize x-ray technology. With that would standardize x-ray technology. With the production of the Techron generator, some radiologists complained to the company that it would be possible for "anyone to take x-ray pictures."

If anyone could do this, what would stop laymen from frivolously making diagnoses? This fear, as much as anything else, may well have driven the science of radiology into the realm of specialization. The words of Dr. Robert Carman, delivered 10 years prior, had proved prophetic.

"The evolution and progress of medical sci-ence and art necessitate division and subdivi-sion of labor — specialization. In medicine, as in everything else, the fewer things a man does, the better he can and ought to do them. The right of a specialty to exist has only this test — that it employ the specialist's entire time and attention with increased benefit to himself, to the profession and to the public. Judged by this test, roentgenology is and of right ought to be a legitimate specialty."

Carman's ideas were heard by more than just physicians. Technicians — like the early radiologists — were beginning to ask, why not

Not All Pioneers Were Bearded

Polish-born Marie Sklodowska was the epitome of a woman destined to fight against the oppression of the time, complet-ing the equivalent of high school, then fur-ther defying what was deemed "ap-propriate" for a young woman by traveling to France alone to further her studies. Enrolling in France's only school offering theoretical physics, Ecole Francaise de Mathematiques, Marie completed her stud-ies at the top of her class. Graduation occurred during a most auspicious time.

The discovery of x-rays had led scientists to further investigate whether rays similar to x-rays could also be produced by ordi-nary fluorescent or phosphorescent sub-stances. French scientist Antoine-Henri Becquerel discovered "spontaneous radia-tion," that is, radiation emanating from cer-tain elements, such as uranium, spon-taneously and persistently.

Marie Sklodowska immediately became interested in this topic and, after her mar-riage to Pierre Curie, began a systematic chemical analysis, eventually discovering a

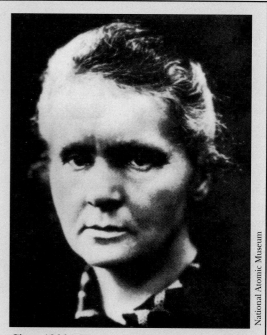

Circa 1900 - Marie Curie

highly radioactive substance emitting 2 mil-lion times as much radiation as uranium. It was called radium, and its discovery was announced in December 1898.

The couple continued to study this new element over the next few years. Noting the "contagious" nature of radium, Madame Curie wrote: "When one studies strongly radioactive substances, special precautions must be taken if one wishes to be able to continue taking delicate measurements.

The various objects used in a chemical laboratory, and those which serve for experiments in physics, all become radioactive in a short time and act upon photographic plates through black paper. Dust, the air of the room, and one's clothes, all become radioactive."

Around 1900 the Curies, intrigued by reports of the destructive action of radium on the skin, began conducting numerous animal experiments, eventually leading to the treatment of patients with Curie therapy. After Pierre's death in 1906, Marie continued to work with radium. In 1911 Marie Curie became the first woman to receive the Nobel Prize in chemistry. That was her second Nobel. In 1903 she shared the prize in physics with her husband and Bequerel.

In 1912 she established the Radium Institute for a variety of research and medical treatments. These were remarkable accomplishments for a woman who was initially denied a college teaching position and had to settle for a menial job at a girl's school.

Marie also offered her services to develop France's medical x-ray facilities and helped set up a mobile radiographic apparatus with a dynamo to supply electricity. As World War I grew fiercer, citizens donated more vehicles to be equipped by her — they became known as "little Curies."

Marie taught herself radiography, driving and auto repair so she wouldn't have to rely on others. She traveled from hospital to hospital, where she spent long hours doing radiologic exams alongside surgeons. Continuing her work with radium after the war, Madame Curie's failure to protect herself from radiation led to her death in 1934 of aplastic anemia. She was 66 years old.

It is interesting to note that Madame Curie's legacy continued to live through her two daughters, Irene and Eve. Irene Joliot-Curie became France's undersecretary of state for scientific research for a brief time. In 1933 she discovered artificial radioactivity. After lecturing at the Sorbonne in 1937, Irene Curie came close to discovering fission, but failed because she did not know how to interpret the results of her research — results which later enabled Otto Hahn to find the true solution to the enigma of the explosion of the uranium nucleus. After World War II, Irene served as director of the Radium Institute, and later was a member of France's Commission for Atomic Energy.

Eve Curie was a World War II correspondent for a number of American newspapers and co-director of the Paris-Presse. She married Henri Labouisse, who served as director general of the United Nations International Children's Emergency Fund (UNICEF). In this capacity, Labouisse went to Stockholm in 1965 to accept the Nobel Peace Prize.

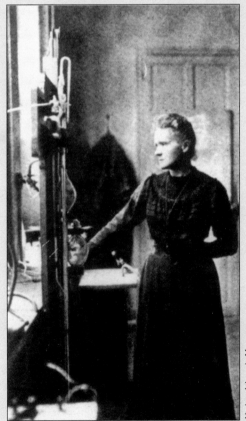

Circa 1903 - *Marie Curie in her laboratory.*

Chapter Three

The Technician's Evangelist

*E*ddy Clifford Jerman (pronounced Ger-man) eventually would be the man to answer the call of the technician's plight. As important as Roentgen was to the discovery of the x-ray and Carman to the specialization of the radiologist, Jerman would be to the development of the technician as a professional. But like many great men and women of science, Jerman came from obscurity — his life shaped by a series of unusual circumstances that would inexorably push him to the forefront of the emerging radiologic technologies.

Born on a small Indiana farm in Ripley County Nov. 21, 1865, to Loda Wick Davis Jerman and Sarah Lucia Lee, Ed Jerman was the eldest of four children. He had a brother, Elmer, born in 1869; a sister, Mary, born in 1878; and another sister, Stella, born in 1880.

Following the Civil War in which he served, Loda Jerman began the study of medicine, attending lectures at the Ohio Medical College of Cincinnati. Medical schools, at this time, were conducted by outstanding physicians of the day, and instruction was given in the form of lectures.

After two years, Dr. Jerman began the practice of medicine, returning to Ohio Medical College eight years later and receiving his diploma in 1879. He would become the exemplary physician — the country doctor. His domain in rural southeastern Indiana was described by his son Elmer as "mostly yellow clay hills, with valley soils being more productive." It was considered by many as "submarginal land," and many farmers in the area sold their holdings for $10 an acre and moved on to greener pastures in Iowa.

Dr. Jerman's home was located four miles from the small town of Batesville, and his practice, typical of the times, required calling on his patients as well as receiving them in his home or at the community center. Since there were no paved roads until the turn of the century, Dr. Jerman made his house calls by horse-drawn buggy.

At the time, people were taxed to improve the roads, but were permitted to work off the tax. Ed Jerman, his brother Elmer and their mother handled the levy by grading up the center of the roads to encourage drainage. During the spring thaws the roads became all but impassable, forcing Dr. Jerman to turn to a two-wheeled gig "with one seat perched high with a box cabinet beneath for his medicine kit," according to Elmer. Dr. Jerman made his calls either with this horse-drawn gig or on horseback.

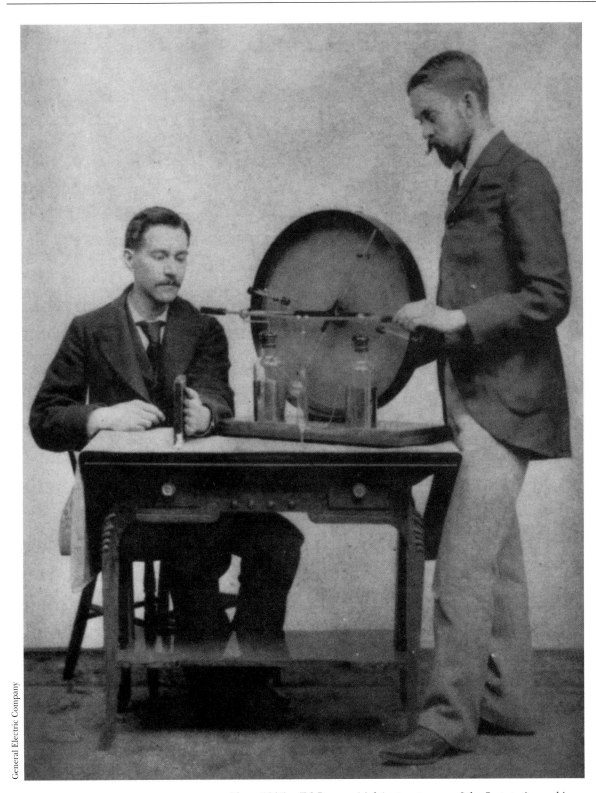

General Electric Company

Circa 1896 - *Ed Jerman (right) operates one of the first static machines.*

Dr. Jerman's medical skill was made available to everyone in the community, regardless of their ability to pay. Epidemics of typhoid fever were common in the area, occurring every fall. Dr. Jerman was regarded as an expert in the treatment of the disease. It was not uncommon for several families in the area to become infected.

Dr. Jerman often made three or four trips a day to the same house to provide treatment, noting each visit on his payment records. After a while he realized that the bill was running too large and began charging for only one trip. This, too, soon became too large. So Jerman stopped charging altogether.

The elder Jerman was active in community politics but never sought an office. According to Elmer, he gave "special attention to the election of township trustees, that he might have, as he once stated, some influence in the selection of teachers for the local school." Jerman also boarded teachers, giving his children the "benefit of their discussions, and many of (the children's) early opinions were formulated thereby."

The Jermans thoroughly believed in education and sacrificed much toward this end. Dr. Jerman's expressed belief was that "he would rather give his children an education than leave them money. They couldn't quarrel over that nor could anyone take it away from them." In pursuit of that education, Dr. Jerman's children first attended a "pioneer country school" — a single-room frame building "perched on top of the clay hills."

Elmer Jerman recalled that as many as 65 to 75 pupils a day attended the school, equipped with "wooden seats placed longitudinally against the sidewalls, and as (we) sat with (our) backs to the wall... (We) often pasted paper over the cracks to keep the cold winds from hitting us." A large wood stove, box pattern, was placed in the center of the room for heat. Water came from a bucket,

complete with tin cups, and "it was a treat to be permitted to go for water."

Ed Jerman in later years would comment that "his instruction in grammar in that very early school was the best thing that happened to him." But these primitive schools that served much of rural America bestowed far more than just grammar. "Character, industry, thrift, self-confidence and self-reliance was imparted to the youth of (this) time through both the home and school."

As important as education was during these days, the influence of home life and community was equally formative for the Jerman children. Because of their father's interest in politics, the two Jerman boys frequently found themselves playing about the polls, and according to an account by Elmer, "often saw a worker take a 'floater' by the arm, put a ticket in his hand and lead him up to the polls where the ticket could be deposited in the box. Nothing much was said about it, except family comments as to the disgrace of selling one's vote, and (we) became convinced as to the evil thereof."

The Jermans were rigid disciplinarians, and Dr. Jerman insisted his children be kept busy. Both Ed and Elmer were in charge of planting the fields with corn and wheat, tending the garden and cutting winter firewood. As a reward, Dr. Jerman permitted his sons to attend the county fair. However, the elder Jerman also had a list of prohibitions — attending dances, playing cards, playing ball on Sunday and, most stringent of all, drinking.

Both Jermans were strong advocates of temperance. Dr. Jerman once told a neighbor that "the only thing that would make him send one of his boys away from home was for that boy to come home drunk." But boys would be boys. Dr. Jerman kept whiskey or peach brandy on hand in his office, and his sons "sampled it" on rare occasion.

Elmer wrote: "On one occasion, we (Ed

and Elmer) took cream pitchers to the cellar and drew from a keg a supply of currant wine which we enjoyed very much. In these early days, Father was accustomed to rolling his own pills, dishing out powders, making ointments, cough syrup, etc. The taste of his cough syrup was pleasing to us, and he kept a bottle in the house. Once, upon his return from a Grange meeting, he noticed the bottle of cough syrup and immediately inquired what had become of it. Of course, we told him, and he administered doses of ipecac, thereby getting rid of the syrup."

Fortunately, such healthy curiosity would eventually begin to direct Ed Jerman's future course. During his elementary school days, Jerman's teacher brought an electric battery to school. While it may have been nothing more than a plaything to the majority of the students, "it meant a lot more to (Ed), since it stirred up a spark of interest that never afterwards faded."

Whether accidental or planned, Dr. Jerman soon after purchased a Faradic battery operated by an acid cell battery and a Jerome Kidder magnetic type battery. As these batteries "occasionally got out of order... and being somewhat of a mechanical turn of mind, (Ed) was permitted to try his hand at repairing them, as there was no service available nearer than Cincinnati."

Ed Jerman was so successful at this, he eventually began performing repairs for other doctors in the area. "They would bring their batteries to (our) home and usually stay until they were repaired. There was never any charge for this work, and board and feed for their horses was also gratis," Jerman wrote. Following these experiences, Jerman attempted to construct an electric light, but without success. Jerman's interest in electricity, however, went undaunted. His first "electrical pay job" was installing a night watchman's detector (a burglar alarm) for the Greeman Brothers Furniture Manufacturing Company in Batesville.

Equipped with a keen mind, an interest in electromechanical apparatus and an upbringing that encouraged education, Ed Jerman left his home and began a journey toward a destiny that would eventually lead him to the x-ray. But more than anything else, it would be Jerman's health that would be both a help and a hindrance.

In 1882 he entered Franklin College in Franklin, Ind., a small town not far from Indianapolis. During his three-year tenure at Franklin, Jerman's interest in experimentation would blossom. After his job in Batesville, Jerman developed and installed a burglar and fire alarm system for a local company, but he failed to patent the device. It was later patented by a New York firm and went on to be widely used.

An example of Jerman's ingenuity, the system used thermostats on an open circuit and thin strips of fusible metal on a closed circuit for the fire alarm system. Similarly, the burglar alarm system consisted of thin strips of metal foil on a closed circuit on window panes and door panels, with the closed circuit linking window and door springs. All circuits were connected to a central station.

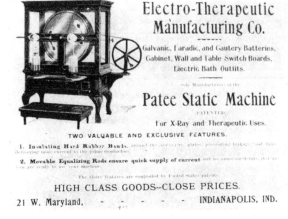

Circa 1900 - An early ad for the Patee Static Machine, made by the Electro-Therapeutic Manufacturing Co.

Jerman's interest in electrical devices was further whetted while attending physics classes. There he first began experimenting with vacuum tubes, including the Geisler and Crookes tubes. His poor health, however, brought about a change in plans, and he was forced to suspend his studies after three years.

Traveling to West Texas in 1885 because of his health, Jerman found work with a Chicago agency selling a book, *Happy Homes and the Hearts That Make Them.* Unfortunately, the books that Jerman ordered became his property. While he had no trouble taking orders, when it came to delivery, many purchasers refused. Jerman later commented, "The people of Texas didn't want happy homes, so this venture proved a failure."

Jerman, however, did not give up. With his health improving, he went to work for H.I. Talley of Austin, Texas, doing electrical wiring, bell hanging and repairing medical batteries. He also attended Austin's Central Business College at night — perhaps realizing his failure as a book salesman was due to a lack of business acumen.

But it wasn't all books and business for Jerman in those days. Six months of his stay in Texas included work as a flyer with a prairie schooner trading expedition from San Antonio into Chihuahua, Mexico, riding horseback and sleeping in the open with a saddle as a pillow for the entire trip. Jerman would later write: "It was my business to provide the party with fresh meat (game). Got my first

> **6**
>
> *All wood used in making this equipment was South American mahogany purchased at 20¢ per pound in the rough. Fifty dollars worth of gold leaf was used in ornamenting the static machine case. Hundreds of galvanic, Faradic and cautery batteries were made in this shop and sold throughout the country.*
>
> **9**

and only bear on this trip, a cub at that." Returning to Indiana rejuvenated and once again in good health, Jerman married Martha Adaline Bloom of Franklin in the fall of 1887. Typical of the time, Jerman, his new bride, his mother and father moved in together. They located in New Point, Ind.

In 1889 Jerman went to work for the Jones Brothers Electric Company of Cincinnati, installing a variety of gas and electrical systems throughout the city. He soon switched employers, moving to Physician's and Surgeon's Supply Company, which brought him one step further to an unforeseen goal. Earning $15 per week, Jerman was made foreman of the company's shop, repairing medical batteries.

In 1891 Jerman was sent to Indianapolis to supervise the wiring of the H.E. Allen Surgical Institute, a 400-room facility. For the next six years Jerman would work out of a basement shop from which "very complete medical electric equipment was made and installed." Included in this equipment was a 16-glass plate static machine, several galvanic and Faradic batteries operated "with sal ammoniac wet cells," a Kellogg Sinusoidal machine, various photo therapy lamps, cautery equipment, various miniature lamp equipment for examination of cavities of the body and numerous electrodes.

Jerman was very proud of his work. He would later write: "All wood used in making this equipment was South American mahogany purchased at 20¢ per pound in the rough. Fifty dollars worth of gold leaf was used in ornamenting the static machine case. Hundreds of galvanic, Faradic and cautery batteries were made in this shop and sold throughout the country."

But this was just the beginning. In 1892 Jerman began manufacturing Patee Static Machines for the inventor, T.H. Patee, of Greencastle, Ind. The machines, built in lots of five or 10, featured a revolving glass plate 18 inches in diameter with one stationary plate 20 inches in diameter enclosed in a case. These machines were sold mainly to lightning rod dealers and agents to illustrate their value as protection from lightning, though, Jerman noted, "A few were sold to Physical Laboratories and occasionally one was sold to a doctor (usually a quack or 'advertising' doctor)."

Everything was in place when Roentgen's discovery was announced. Jerman read the newspaper reports and, later, the accounts in scientific journals. Realizing that he had all the necessary equipment to duplicate the experiments with the exception of a Crookes tube, Jerman immediately ordered one. The tube arrived, and on the evening of March 16, 1896, his experiments started.

According to Jerman, "There were present at this party Dr. C.M. Sawyer; Mr. James McGowan, superintendent of the Allen Surgical Institute; Mr. Leonard Curtis; and Mr. W.B. Foster. Curtis and Foster turned the crank of the machine one at a time as they would tire of the job. The party ended at 3:00, the next morning. The usual exposure of keys and coins were made and finally a hand was exposed. The hand was bound to the plate and table with electrical adhesive tape and the exposure was of thirty minutes duration. After about one-half hour spent in developing the plate and with a slight stretch of the imagination, the shadow of the bones of the fingers might be seen."

Enough of a stretch, it would seem, to ignite Jerman's imagination. Jerman the salesman, the electrician, the experimenter, was soon to become the independent businessman and lecturer. Obtaining the exclusive rights to the Patee Static Machine, Jerman organized the Electro-Therapeutic Manufacturing Company and moved to Indianapolis. The company made and sold various kinds of medical electrical equipment as well as the static machines.

Jerman was in charge of installing this variety of equipment, as well as delivering instructions on its use. During this period Jerman first made contact with the Victor Electric Company. Victor motors and mechanical speed controllers were used almost exclusively to operate much of the equipment manufactured by Jerman.

In 1897 Jerman imported nearly 200 vacuum tubes from England and Belgium. Some were made of "uranium glass, some of lead glass, and others of flint glass. Some of them contained various gasses and some fluorescent combinations. Some consisted of a tube within a tube, the inner vacuum tube being surrounded with various solutions, such as sulphate of copper, sulphate of quinine and potassium bichromate."

Jerman used these tubes in more than 100 lectures delivered to students throughout Indiana to demonstrate the effect of "the passing of high volume electric current through vacuums of various degrees (and) through various gas mediums." For the next 10 years Jerman presented six to 12 lectures each school year, discussing medical electricity and the x-ray, during which time he provided demonstrations of the equipment.

In 1902 the Electro-Therapeutic Manufacturing Company failed, "due to the secretary and general manager absconding with all available cash and through general mismanagement. It was found that he had been secretly withdrawing funds for his own use over a period of a year or more." Left without "a dollar in reserve," Jerman continued to do service and repair work until 1903, at which time his health again took a downward turn.

Once again, however, Jerman's poor physical health brought positive results. Leaving his family behind, Jerman headed for La Junta, Colo., but only made it as far as Topeka, Kan., before illness cut short his trip. He quickly became acquainted with a group of physicians and surgeons, who "gave friendly council, advice and treatment as well as some x-ray work to do." Within eight months Jerman recovered, gained 20 pounds and reached the decision that Topeka was "a good enough place to live."

After relocating his family to Topeka, Jerman made another abortive attempt at establishing his own business. In 1904 he formed a small company, again manufacturing the static machines. The company was later incorporated into the National X-Ray Company and remained prosperous for nearly eight years. One reason for the prosperity was Jerman's association with Schiedel Western Company, which chose him as exclusive agent for the company's coil, the Schiedel Western 16-inch Radiographic Special, and later the Schiedel Western Premier, Peerless and Universal transformers.

While Jerman was busy selling and installing this equipment, bankruptcy befell the manager of the National X-Ray Company. For a second time, Jerman found himself financially stranded. He continued to work as a sales agent for Schiedel Western, a position he held until the company merged with Victor Electric, the Snook Roentgen Company and the Macalaster Wiggin Company in 1916.

Jerman was then 51 years old, and the weight of failure was becoming oppressive. His oldest daughter had died in 1910 and his father, who had provided so much inspiration, passed away in 1915. The responsibilities to his wife, Ada, his mother and his remaining daughter, Lucile, and two grandchildren, Edna and Marie, drove Jerman toward a mental crisis during which he contemplated giving up his life's work and entering a new field of endeavor.

Jerman lamented, "In an earnest and extended effort to analyze my own situation

past, present and future, several facts regarding the situation became apparent. I consulted freely with many of my x-ray friends from various companies and from various parts of the country in an effort to clarify the situation. I had worked conscientiously to the extent of my physical ability but had only succeeded in making a scanty living, and at times, hardly that. I was only able to provide for my family the barest necessities."

The conclusions that Jerman ultimately reached regarding his life provide an insight into the methodology used by many of the traveling x-ray salesmen of the day. Many of his competitors received a commission of between 30 and 40 percent of a sale, which could range between $1,500 and $10,000. Sale and installation of the equipment generally took two days. One of Jerman's competitors admitted that to make a sale he would recommend that the doctor "employ Jerman to give you the instruction and you will get the results and save some money as well."

Responding to these types of leads, Jerman received between $25 and $50 for a week's instruction, but paid his own expenses. Recognizing the flaw in this design, Jerman visited one his most active competitors and posed the question: "I work more hours than you do. I have been at the work much longer than you have. I believe that I know as much about the work as you do. What's wrong with me?"

Fortunately for Jerman, he received a candid reply. "You sell a man equipment and then spend a week to ten days teaching him how to use it. You go back from time to time to help him, spending your money for the time and expenses. I sell a man an outfit and following its arrival I install it, get my settlement and leave. While you are instructing and following up on your customer, I am getting two or three more orders.

"Your method has one advantage in my favor: you cannot cover a large territory. I cannot successfully meet your kind of competition, and really don't try very hard. I have plenty of territory outside of yours to work." Jerman's territory, at the time, included Kansas, outside of the river towns (mainly the Kansas City area). His competitor covered not only Kansas, but several surrounding states as well.

Caught between conscience and calamity, Jerman gave up his quest. But after three months, he decided to invest what little was left of his savings in visiting "a number of my x-ray friends in various parts of the country in a search for further light." The trip was propitious. During each visit, Jerman took copious notes.

Whenever an x-ray operator was found doing something exceptionally well, Jerman would inquire as to how the method had been

developed. Often he was met with the reply: "That's my secret. You'll have to find out, as I did, by practice and experience." Others would attempt to explain their "technic," but their skill had been acquired in such a way that they were "unable to impart much information of value."

Jerman's frustration was evident. He wrote: "It was difficult to find two operators who were anywhere near in accord regarding technical procedure. Some would advise certain procedures and others entirely different procedures. The utmost confusion regarding technical procedure existed. The great variety of equipment only added to the confusion."

Despondent, Jerman returned home and actually considered "depositing the notes in the stove, but for some unaccountable reason put them on a nearby table instead." Two

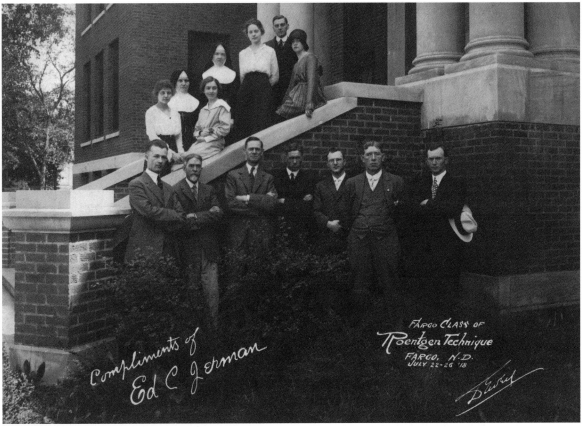

In 1917 the Victor X-Ray Company hired Ed Jerman to head its education department. Jerman, second from the left on the bottom row, autographed this photo for the members of a class he taught in Fargo, N.D., in 1918.

weeks later Jerman revisited these notes. He later wrote: "About midnight a vision in the form of a new light regarding the situation appeared." Jerman's vision was both simple and imminently practical.

Jerman wrote: "All men interested in x-ray work — the manufacturer, the salesman, the technician and the doctor should be intensely interested in the end results, the bringing about of the best possible result for the patient. This result should fully justify the total investment of time, labor and material involved. Three great essentials are involved in the success or failure of any x-ray laboratory — equipment, technique and interpretation. Any handicap with either or any of these essentials can only contribute towards failure."

Jerman knew there was a vast amount of quality x-ray equipment available, and that rapid strides were being made in the continuing improvement of this equipment. He also concluded that the doctor, with his knowledge of anatomy and pathology, could quickly begin to acquire valuable information from good plates, if good plates were available. A few medical schools and radiologists at the time were providing some instruction regarding interpretation.

But accurate, reliable instruction regarding technique was nowhere available.

Reaching this conclusion, Jerman wrote: "Evidently the weakest link of the chain was technique, and the chain could be no stronger than its weakest link. The manufacturer and doctor must be interested in strengthening this link." Jerman decided to step into this breach and "devote the rest of my life work in an effort toward strengthening this link, fully realizing the immense size of the problem and many of the vast difficulties and prejudices to be overcome. It looked like a real man-sized job."

It was indeed, and the first discouraging

results would have daunted a man with less conviction than Jerman. Medical schools and universities had "no room or time for such work." Jerman then decided to approach manufacturers, hoping one would agree to establish an educational department. His first visit was to the Victor X-Ray Company, where his ideas were met with guarded optimism. Such a plan, he was advised, might be considered in the future.

Jerman pressed forward. He contacted several of the Victor representatives with an appeal for their support, hoping to find doctors with x-ray equipment who would pay $100 for a week's private instruction in x-ray technique. Again Jerman met with resistance.

"It was argued that the doctors would never consent to paying such a price. I argued that there were a great many doctors with x-ray equipment of from $3,000 to $10,000 who were obtaining but a small part of the results, possibly due mainly to their lack of technical knowledge or skill. That if the doctor should even invest $500 for such training and thereby (be) enabled to improve his results to the extent of from 1 to 500 percent, this investment would prove the most profitable part of his entire investment."

Two Victor representatives responded to Jerman's appeal, a Mr. Lewis located in Des Moines, Iowa, and Dr. Ingersoll in Los Angeles. Choosing Lewis, whose territory encompassed Chicago, Jerman waited. After six weeks Lewis reported that he had been unable to sell the idea to anyone.

Jerman wrote back to Lewis, asking him to make a week's date with someone in Des Moines for "$100, $50, $25, or, if necessary, no charge at all." Such was Jerman's faith in the idea. "If (we) could not give it away, we would pay someone for the privilege of delivering a trial week's instruction."

The gamble paid off. A Dr. Lear of Des Moines agreed to pay $50 — "if he felt, at the end of the week, that he had received value to that extent."

Jerman delivered the week's instruction, working seven straight days at Mercy Hospital in Des Moines. At the end of the week, Dr. Lear paid Jerman $100, saying, "You do not have to reduce your price for me, as I have received value in full for the entire amount at the end of the first two days' work." In addition, Lewis and Dr. Lear succeeded in making three more appointments before the week was over. Jerman would remain in Iowa for a year, and his fee would rise to $150, plus expenses, for six days' work.

The relationship between Jerman and Lewis was beneficial to them both. Jerman at last was working steadily, following his vision. Lewis, because of his association with Jerman, was also reaping financial rewards. Jerman wrote: "Everywhere I went, orders for accessories and additional equipment quickly followed. (Lewis') volume of business more than doubled over that of the previous year. I received greater remuneration for my services than I had ever received before."

Success was at hand. In what may have been Jerman's first true class in "technic," 10 students attended from the Des Moines area. It was not without incident. Jerman wrote: "A patient was in a lateral knee position on the table, with the tube placed crosswise with the table. Two or three of the students were standing at the switchboard, one of them operating the machine. The machine was started and the patient's knee slipped out of position.

"I motioned the operator to wait a moment and proceeded to reposition the patient, standing with my forehead an inch or so from the terminal of the tube with my hands on the metal table. The operator thoughtlessly closed the x-ray switch. When I came to I found myself on a couch with the group surrounding me, a knob the size of a small hen's egg on my forehead, (and) a quite pro-

nounced smell of burnt hair. Within fifteen or twenty minutes the evening's work proceeded as though nothing had happened. It was many weeks, however, before I fully recovered from the effects of the shock."

Undaunted by such accidents, Jerman pressed forward, and news of his success began to circulate. He received visits from representatives of the General Electric Company — manufacturer of the Coolidge tube that Jerman was using — and the Eastman Kodak Company. Both representatives offered Jerman jobs demonstrating their respective products. Jerman declined. He was after bigger game. "I had my heart set on the Victor X-Ray Company," he wrote, "and decided I would eventually get what I was after or continue to work alone."

His wait was short. In 1917 Victor sent a visiting auditor to witness Jerman's work. Within a short time after this, Jerman was again visited and offered a position. On May 20, 1917, Victor established its Educational Department with Jerman as its head. A "red-letter day" in his life, Jerman wrote: "One of the most valuable lessons of this 52 years of life was: First be sure you are right in having a perfectly feasible vision, then with patience, perseverance and hard work you are most certain to win. Nothing can stop honest, conscientious, intelligent and continued effort but physical inability or death."

Indeed, Eddy Clifford Jerman had a perfectly feasible vision, and with success came an apparent need that this vision be extended.

> '
> *I motioned the operator to wait a moment and proceeded to reposition the patient, standing with my forehead an inch or so from the terminal of the tube with my hands on the metal table. The operator thoughtlessly closed the x-ray switch.*
> '

The Better the Technology, The Better the Technician

In the early part of the century, the biggest complaint of technicians with even the best understanding of their equipment was the inability to exactly duplicate x-ray studies. Consistent exposures were nearly impossible, given low current, varying voltage and differing degrees of vacuum from tube to tube. But help was on the way.

In 1907 Philadelphia physicist and x-ray equipment manufacturer Homer Clyde Snook — one of the few nonmedical members admitted to the ARRS — installed his "interrupterless transformer" in Jefferson Hospital, Philadelphia. Snook used a direct current motor and applied a rotary converter to change to alternating current, then mounted a rectifying switch on the converter shaft, which locked the switch to the AC cycle and ensured that only the negative phase of the current would be fed into the cathode of the tube.

Snook also replaced the conventional induction coil with a much more efficient closed magnetic circuit transformer with minimal magnetic leakage, sealed in an oil-filled tank. He added a rheostat for varying the current continuously, thus allowing voltage and amperage to be controlled. In essence, the power source was now capable of producing quality x-rays. Snook's apparatus won immediate approval and would remain the standard for the next 10 years.

But the power source was only a part of the problem. The Fleming valve used on the Snook apparatus was inherently unstable because of residual gas in the valve. This problem was overcome in 1914 by Saul Dushman of General Electric, who developed the Kenetron, a new rectifier tube. The Kenetron was a hot-cathode Fleming valve from which almost all of the gas had been evacuated. Although early models produced only slight improvements, further experimentation resulted in the design of a Kenetron that met all x-ray requirements and became widely used.

William Coolidge, also of General Electric, developed models of the hot-cathode tube (a self-rectifying tube), which simplified the equipment, as well as making it safer. Enclosed in the same metal container with the transformer, the tube opened the way for the construction of a portable x-ray unit with a capacity of 85 kVp and 10 mA.

Refinements continued, and by the

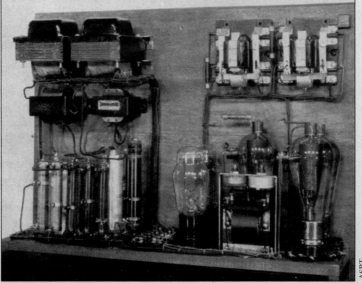

Circa 1936 - *An early electronic impulse x-ray timer.*

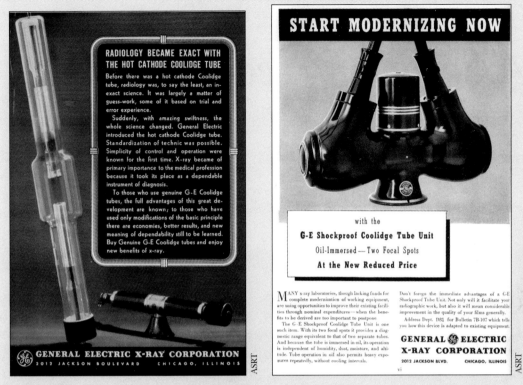

Shown above are two examples of ads in the X-Ray Technician *that were run by GE: The Hot Cathode Coolidge Tube (left) and the Shockproof Coolidge Tube (right).*

1950s die-hard rivals Kodak and Du Pont had significantly improved x-ray film sensitivity and speed. Automatic film processors revolutionized darkroom methods in the mid-50s. The electronic image intensifier was considered an instant boon, as was the ultra-speed Roentgen motion picture unit (known as the Micronex), capable of one-millionth of a second high intensity x-ray exposures.

Teaching methods also began to be modernized. A plastic model of a standard x-ray unit was completed in 1950, in which colored plastics were lit electronically in such a manner that the internal workings could be demonstrated in a simplified manner. The model, however, was costly — $3,600. So a series of color slides were produced, along with a motion picture showing the model in operation.

Chapter Four

A Society of Technicians

*E*d Jerman's guiding principles and goals were not compromised by his association with the Victor X-Ray Company. If anything, it became an extremely positive symbiotic relationship in which Victor enjoyed increased sales of equipment as a direct result of Jerman's educational programs, and Jerman had the opportunity to expand his teaching to a much wider group of radiologists and technicians. Jerman, however, inheriting his father's political beliefs, began to envision a larger goal.

With his financial woes at last laid to rest and in relatively good health, Jerman was confronted with an ethical question: how best to organize a group that would contribute to the development of the technician's stature in radiology. The most common type of organization sweeping America at the time was the labor union, and many technicians favored such a structure as a means to collectively enhance their working conditions and pay scale.

Jerman, however, was strongly opposed to unionization, perhaps because he understood the perspective of radiologists regarding technicians. A heavy-handed approach to organization surely would have disastrous results. Additionally, many of the technicians with whom Jerman came into contact were

Catholic Sisters. It was apparent what was needed was a professional society that would be acceptable to all.

Also, as a charter member of ARRS, Jerman was aware of the threat from several states considering legislation that would impose undesired regulations and restrictions on technicians. The need to create a national organization preemptive of such legislation became imperative. With the war in Europe now over and the prosperity of the Roaring '20s about to reshape America, Jerman's timing was excellent.

On Oct. 25, 1920, Jerman brought together a group of 13 technicians from nine states and one province of Canada for the purpose of organizing a society of x-ray technicians. In attendance were Glenn Files of Chicago; Carl Reed of Minneapolis; Herbert H. Newman of Tampa, Fla.; W.H. Thompson of Mobile, Ala.; H.O. Mahoney of Duluth, Minn.; C.J. Bodle of Winnipeg, Canada; Mrs. S. Christofferson of Portland, Ore.; Freda Copple of Kansas City, Mo.; Jessie Gordon of St. Joseph, Mo.; Marie K. MacDonald of Des Moines, Iowa; Ruth Thoroman of Newton, Iowa; Alma O. Carlson of Minneapolis; and P.J. Blegan of Webster, S.D.

Conducted in the offices of the Victor

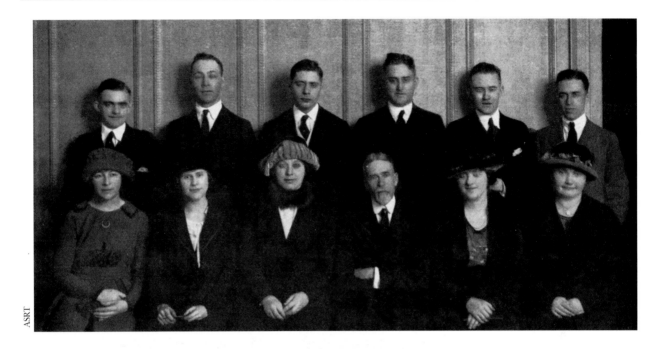

ASRT

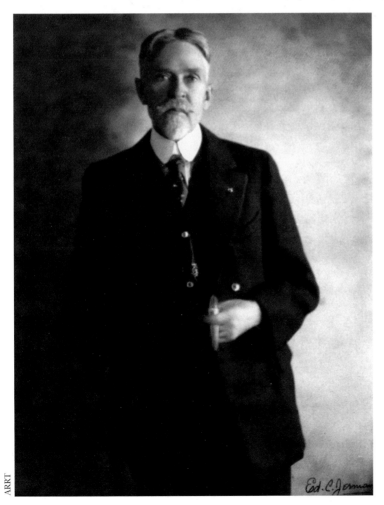

ARRT

Circa 1920 - *(top)*
Twelve of the first 14 members of what
became the ASRT.

1865-1936 – *Ed C. Jerman (left)*

X-Ray Company, Jerman's meeting also included radiologists and representatives from other x-ray manufacturers. Although neither Jerman nor his subsequent biographers offered an explanation as to how the 13 individuals were selected, logic dictates that these charter members were chosen for a number of reasons.

First, Glenn Files, who later became manager of the technical department of the General Electric X-Ray Corporation, practically had been raised by Jerman. H.O. Mahoney was a technical instructor at General Electric. Carl W. Reed was a technical advisor for the Pengelly X-Ray Company of Minneapolis. These were people on the move in the profession.

Secondly, the remainder of the group represented a geographically diverse lot, perhaps indicative of Jerman's master plan for the association he was forming. The enduring strength of the national association would be built by organizing and supporting state societies. Jerman obviously hoped such encouragement eventually would be passed along to the national Society.

Indeed, other than adopting a constitution and bylaws for the new association, Jerman stressed the importance of "spreading the news." At this first meeting, he appointed state delegates, "whose duty it was to interest technicians in the newly organized association and to promote the object for which the association stood."

Christened the American Association of Radiological Technicians (AART), Jerman was elected president, Carlson as first vice-president, Christofferson as second vice president, Copple as secretary and Thompson as treasurer.

Following the business meeting, brief talks were given by many of the members. Jerman "sought to develop a professional code of ethics" among the technicians at the first meeting. He was quoted as talking "at length

on the work of the Society and advocated high ideals of loyalty to the profession and to the radiologists." Those physicians present not only "voiced their approval of the organization, but gave short addresses of a technical nature. Danger in the use of x-ray and the importance of self-protection were stressed."

Within the AART's constitution, membership was proscribed in several levels. Full membership required that the individual "have devoted the major portion of their time for a period of at least two years, to doing radiological technical work, under the direct supervision or through being associated with regular professional men (referring to recognized radiologists, physicians or surgeons)." Annual dues were set at $5.

Members-elect were required to have served at least one year in radiologic technical work, with annual dues set at $2.50. Associate members, with annual dues set at $1, were defined as "individuals who are in any way interested in the use of the x-ray and its application to medicine, science or industry." Finally, honorary members, who paid no dues, were individuals who "distinguished themselves in some branch of radiological research work." Only full members were allowed to vote and hold office in the association.

By the end of the second day of the meeting, the group agreed to meet again in June of the following year, holding open the charter. "Each member was urged to persuade technicians who could meet the qualifications to become charter members" during the 1921 meeting. From that Chicago session, it was noted that the total amount collected for registration and dues — fees for attending the meetings were equivalent to dues — was $120; disbursements and incidental expenses ran $25, leaving a balance of $95, which was turned over to the treasurer.

The meeting concluded and during the following eight months the officers and members "carried on an enthusiastic campaign which spread the good news throughout the country... Many letters of invitation were sent to eligible x-ray technicians in the United States and Canada, inviting them to attend the 1921 meeting and to become charter members."

Jerman's quest for technician credibility had begun, but the road ahead would not be without difficulty. The radiologists, who for so long had battled for their own credibility, were not long in responding to the formation of the AART. Of utmost concern to both the RSNA and ARRS was some method of certification for technicians, and hardly three months after the AART's organizational meeting, the subject was broached at the annual meeting of the RSNA.

Perhaps driven by the same forces that compelled Jerman to establish the AART, the two national radiologist societies suddenly found themselves facing the proverbial "cat out of the bag." As difficult as it had been to gain proper recognition from the AMA, the necessity of maintaining credibility in their own profession, through their technicians, required an immediate response.

Anticipating the success of Jerman's association, a joint committee of the RSNA and ARRS met and decided that some form of recognition of x-ray technicians should be established. The result of the meeting concluded that a technician Registry be established to certify technicians meeting certain qualifications. It took two more years, however, before a consensus was reached concerning these qualifications.

Certainly Jerman anticipated such a response from the RSNA and ARRS, but whether his stature in the radiologic community had any sway over the decisions of those organizations remains unknown. It would soon become apparent, though, that his timing in creating the AART was politically impeccable.

The momentum initiated during that first organizational meeting soon proved undeniable.

On June 27, 1921, the AART's first annual meeting convened for a four-day session in Chicago, again hosted at the Victor X-Ray Company. Thirty-three charter members joined the original 13. Twenty-two individuals were present for the opening session. Perhaps even more impressive was that the charter members represented 18 states and five Canadian provinces.

During the final day of the meeting, the group met at the Morrison Hotel "where the association paid $15 for the use of a meeting room." The morning session "consisted of the presentation of papers by members... dealing with their various problems and technical procedures." At the business session in the afternoon, it was voted to close the charter and set the second annual meeting for Minneapolis in May 1922.

Unfortunately, that meeting was not to be, nor would the AART officially convene again until 1926. What transpired during those four years remains something of a mystery.

In *The Trail of the Invisible Light*, Dr. E.R.N. Grigg suggests the technicians' meetings were suspended on "commercially competitive" grounds. In other words, radiologists were concerned about the motives of the x-ray technicians.

The radiologists' fear of a technicians' organization came at a time when many technicians who had learned their craft at the hands of physicians sought to establish their own credibility. As technicians assumed increased responsibilities and learned new techniques, radiologists worried that they might establish competing clinics for x-ray services and attempt diagnosis without the input of a trained physician.

While the organization exhibited no outward activity for nearly four years, the stimulus from the first two meetings compelled individual technicians to carry on the work and look toward the day when "the ideals inspired by Mr. Jerman might become attainable."

In the meantime, radiologists who favored formal training of x-ray technicians sought facilities for adequate technical education "and recognized the need for some form of control over them to reduce lay interference in the practice of radiology."

What exactly was this lay interference? More than likely, it came in two forms. First were the rogue x-ray laboratories operated by individuals not recognized by the national radiological organizations. The second form of interference came down to more a matter of employee loyalty.

> *It was feared... that the creation of a consciousness of existence among the technicians would lead to a group effort and eventual unionism, and that the elevation of a technician, especially a male technician, to any level of recognition would precipitate the wholesale establishment of lay laboratories in competition with the qualified radiologists.*

Alfred B. Greene, who would later serve as executive secretary of the American Registry of Radiological Technicians, noted in his *History of the Registry*, "It was feared... that the creation of a consciousness of existence among the technicians would lead to a group effort and eventual unionism, and that the elevation of a technician, especially a male technician, to any level of recognition would precipitate the wholesale establishment of lay laboratories in competition with the qualified radiologists."

He continued, "Individuals in the State of California were particularly firm in this conviction, adding that even though the Registry did not approve of lay independence, and would not permit it among registered technicians, there was no way to deprive a technician of his certificate once he got it, even though he were ousted from the Registry, and he could still display it as a decoy in his own private laboratory."

Twenty years later, in 1944, the Registry noted, "That of the 1,100 lay laboratories listed a few years ago, not a single one was operated by a registered technician, although several were run by registered nurses."

The Registry's paranoia was not without basis. A letter written that year by a member of the Registry Board in reply to an inquiry by a technician read:

"...I notice that your name is placed on the letterhead without any doctor's name as being in charge of the department. Are you making the diagnoses and prescribing treatment for a department of the size you mention? If so, I think you are undertaking a great deal of responsibility; and your salary should be about $6,000 a year if your experience warrants your holding such a position. However, we do not contemplate having a technician undertake such responsibilities. In fact, we have put ourselves definitely on record to the contrary. For your protection, and the protection of the clinic, it seems that they should have a physician experienced in roentgenology in charge of the department."

The second impediment, more subtle, actually had nothing to do with lay interference, but came from the radiologists themselves who were confronted with faithful employees attempting to organize. There can be no doubt that the vast majority of technicians in the x-ray workplace were women, and female assertiveness during the 1920s was dimly viewed, especially by the male radiologists who had invested no small amount of time in training their assistants. If the doctor said "no" to the employee's membership in the technicians' society, the job loyalties of the day demanded that the female employee obey his orders, an entrenched view that remained steadfast for the next four decades.

Such prohibition by radiologists was evident, even in the makeup of the AART. Of those charter members of the Society, the division between male and female was almost equal — 23 men, 21 women — certainly not an accurate representation of the total technician workforce throughout the United States and Canada.

But there were further complications, as would soon be discovered by the joint committee of the RSNA and ARRS studying the feasibility of creating a Registry for technicians. According to Greene, "The American Registry of X-Ray Technicians was not an accident. It came into being as the brain-child of a group of wise and far-seeing radiologists who saw in the future the need for a skill and artistry and fidelity in x-ray that far exceeded Roentgen's modest dreams."

But before the Registry could be established, two problems had to be solved. The first was that the Registry would be subject to RSNA's jurisdiction in handling Registry funds; therefore, the RSNA was legally responsible for the acts of the Registry Board. Legal parameters were set and the Registry was established as its own distinct entity, separate from yet sponsored by the RSNA.

The second sticking point dealt with standards of education. Other than Jerman's hands-on teachings, no formal educational programs existed for technicians within the medical community. Whether Jerman played a role in the eventual standards accepted by the Registry remains unknown, but his emergence as the Registry's first examiner hints that for the four years during which the AART did not meet, Jerman was busy behind the scenes, fighting for recognition of not only technicians and the AART, but also for formal education programs.

The American Registry of Radiological Technicians (ARRT) officially came into being early in 1923 — although certification began on Nov. 18, 1922. Application standards and examinations were arranged for prospects. The registration fee was set at $10, with a provision for an additional $1 each time the applicant repeated the examination. Letters explaining the Registry and its process were sent to members of all the radiologist societies.

Those early applications reflected the sense of urgency felt by the radiologist societies to establish something that would pass for an acceptable registration. Better than nothing, "the early blanks were quite brief and requested only very sketchy information about the applicant," according to Greene. No attempt was made to check up on the truthfulness of the responses; and it was "rumored" that occasional certificates were issued simply upon receipt of an application and fee, "although there is no hard evidence to support this unkind reflection upon the integrity of the pioneering members of the Registry."

The first examinations consisted of 50 questions, all of which had to be answered. Two percent was given for each correct answer, and 60 percent was required for passage. Because the Registry was a new enterprise, accurate records were not kept, making it difficult to ascertain precisely who the first registered technician was. Among the first was Helene MacCloude, technician to Dr. A.F. Tyler, who coincidentally was at the time president of RSNA. A certificate was also issued to Glenn Files in 1923, "showing him to be among the pioneers."

Historical records of the AART, however, indicate Sister Mary Beatrice Merrigan of Oklahoma City probably was the first technician to take the Registry examination.

Many of the questions on Sister Mary Beatrice's exam still would be applicable today. A few examples include: "In what way does x-ray

Member Number 77

Edward Gunson was a 19-year-old orphan in 1925 when he approached his uncle, a dentist, for advice on choosing a career. The uncle prided himself on keeping current in his profession and subscribed to all the major medical journals of the day. He had been following with interest the

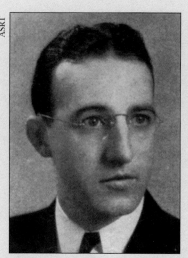

Circa 1936 - Edward Gunson

boom in x-ray technology and thought his young nephew might fit into that world. Edward, after all, had a strong mechanical bent and enjoyed math and science.

Edward's uncle called upon some associates at Strong Memorial Hospital in nearby Rochester, New York, who interviewed Edward and in 1926 agreed to accept him as the first student in their x-ray department. Under the tutelage of the only other member of the department, William Hill, Edward learned to master the equipment, even though nurses performed the majority of the x-ray work.

Gunson ate all his meals at the hospital and in between exams would mop the floors and fold linen. After one year at the hospital, he decided he was ready to become a full-fledged x-ray technician. The year was 1928, and Gunson wrote: "there was no formal graduation ceremony or official certificate edged in gilt. There wasn't even a party. William Hill just came up to me one day and told me it was time for me to begin performing the exams by myself."

Gunson began working 12 hours a day, six days a week, taking an average of 20 x-rays each day. In return, he was paid $100 a month — slightly more than 30 cents an hour. "Pay was never a reason to enter this profession," Gunson said. "After I became an instructor in the '60s, I told my students that they were never going to get rich from this career, so they'd better be darn sure they at least enjoyed it."

Not all the physicians with whom Gunson had contact supported technicians. One, however, encouraged him to become registered. "I took my Registry exam in 1928 while sitting at the desk in my office. I had to write an essay, answer a couple of oral questions and submit 10 or 12 samples of my work. I was thrilled when I received notice that I had passed the exam, because there were only two or three registered x-ray technicians in the entire Rochester area at the time. I felt like I was a member of a terribly exclusive club!"

In 1929 Gunson left Strong Memorial Hospital and took a position at Rochester General Hospital. While there he heard the other x-ray technicians talking about a man named Ed Jerman and the society he had created. Some of the technicians were eager to join the new society, but others called it a move toward unionization and refused to have anything to do with it.

Gunson thought long and hard about whether to join. "I talked to my old teacher, William Hill, and asked him what he thought of the new society," he said. "He told me it would never amount to anything because there was no way the physicians were going to support it. So I decided right then and there that I wanted to be a member."

Gunson became AART member number 77, a distinction that he wore with pride throughout the rest of his career. Gunson went on to publish more than a dozen research papers, serve as president of his local and state technologist societies and deliver the New York Society's 1965 Arthur W. Fuchs Memorial Lecture. He retired from his position as an instructor of radiologic technology at Genessee General Hospital in Rochester.

But the highlight of his career was being among the first group of technicians to be elevated to Fellow status in the national society. "I was elevated to Fellow in 1956, the same year as John Cahoon, Sister Mary Beatrice Merrigan and Edward White — the real pioneers of the profession." When presented with the suggestion that he, too, was a pioneer, Gunson shook his head in wonder and said, "Pioneer? Me? I was just doing my job."

Gunson died Jan. 29, 1995, at the age of 90.

— *Ceela McElveny*

energy differ from light energy?", "What is the difference between primary, secondary and stray or indifferent radiation?" and "When making an x-ray of the hip, in what position should you keep the foot and how would you do it?"

Although these questions may seem fairly straight-forward to the radiologic science student of today, keep in mind that Sister Mary Beatrice did not have access to formal classes or textbooks because there weren't any. In addition to her written answers, the Sister also had to submit sample films of the hand, knee, shoulder, mastoid, frontal sinus, chest, pelvis, kidney, stomach and one full set of dental films. She received a letter from the Registry Board dated Dec. 26, 1922, notifying her of success in passage of the examination. She received her certificate of registration in 1923.

The following year brought significant change for the Registry. Dr. Edward C. Rowe was named president; Dr. Byron C. Darling, vice president; and Dr. E.S. Blaine, secretary. Jerman was reappointed examiner. As Greene later wrote, "There was some opposition from the start to Mr. Jerman's association with the Registry Board because of his connections with the commercial field, but investigation revealed that his work with the Registry, for which his qualifications pre-eminently fitted him, were not biased by his business affiliations."

Had the Registry and the AART at last come to terms? Perhaps not completely, but strides were being made in validation and cooperation. The number of examination questions was reduced from 50 to 10. "Serial numbers were assigned to applicants and the examinations were graded by these numbers, without reference to the individual," to eliminate the "personal element." This was later discontinued.

As the number of registered technicians increased, "the evidence of superior qualifications became associated with preference for employment in the minds of some radiologists. It progressed to the point to which registered technicians were offered free classified advertising in *Radiology* for the purpose of securing positions, although the recommendation was made that the Registry collect a fee of ten to twenty dollars from technicians who secured employment through these channels."

During its first full year (1922-1923), the Registry reported a total of 89 individuals passing its examination. By 1925 the number of registered technicians had grown to 290. That same year, at a meeting of the ARRS, officers of the AART and the Registry met and agreed to restrict membership in the national professional association to registered technicians. Members of the AART were notified they should seek registration or they would automatically be dropped from the roster. All but one promptly achieved registration.

It was a significant move to promote a higher degree of technical expertise and ethical standards into an occupation searching for professional status. As the country inexorably moved toward the Great Depression, this effort would not become easier.

In April 1926 the AART re-emerged as a viable entity, holding a reorganization meeting at the LaSalle Hotel in Chicago. Twelve new members were present, seven of whom were women. Also of significance was the organization of regional associations. The first such society, the Twin Cities Society of X-Ray Technicians, was formed in Minnesota in 1922. In 1924 the King County Technicians Society (of Washington State) was organized. They were joined in 1926 by the Chicago Society and the St. Louis Society of X-Ray Technicians.

The AART reorganization meeting, which lasted three days, dealt mainly with problems that had arisen in the years since the last meeting, particularly those concerning professionalism. Perhaps because of his experiences with the Registry, Jerman suggested changes in the bylaws, discontinuing the category of associate membership and thereby eliminating any non-technicians from the organization. He also suggested that application for any grade of membership, except honorary, require that the applicant be in good standing with his local organization or be endorsed by two good-standing members of the association.

The meeting adjourned and Jerman, obviously satisfied with the progress made, prepared to embark upon what would be the first of many international trips to spread the gospel of "technic." During a two-year period, Jerman and his daughter, Lucile Harwood, traveled to Australia and Europe. By the time

he returned to the United States, 79 new names had been added to the AART's membership roster — now 116 strong.

The Registry, too, was making advancements. In 1927 the Registry decided to canvas radiologists to determine whether they were still in favor of the organization. A questionnaire was prepared and mailed, asking for "frank and detailed opinion(s) concerning the continuation of the Registry as a project, and of its policies and procedures in particular. Of 322 responses, 302 favored continuance of the Registry, with only three additional having any changes to suggest in the manner of procedure."

The remaining 17 were forcefully against the Registry. One radiologist commented that "this Registry of Technicians is the most harmful thing that can be done for the future peace of the radiologists. You have simply formed a Society of people to advance their own interests and eventually fight us... If any of my six technicians joined it they would be looking for a new job!"

Also at this time an analysis was made of the Registry's rolls. It was found that of the 432 registered technicians, 80 or about 18 percent, were men. Of the remaining 82 percent of women, 64 percent were nurses, comprising about 52 percent of the total registration. The figures showed that 153 Sisters were registered, representing 43 percent of the female group and 35 percent of the entire registration.

The study also revealed some interesting facts on the registered technologists' geographic distribution. The Central and Southern portions of the United States contributed most, while the East and West made a "fair showing in spite of the preponderance of opposition coming from these directions."

It appeared that both the AART and the Registry were finally coming of age. Their growth was part of a larger picture that shaped not only these organizations, but the people behind them. What was the world like in the years 1920-1927?

In the United States, the Roaring '20s began with passage of the Volstead Act — Prohibition. Tetraethyl lead anti-knock gasoline went on the market. Bathing beauties' "costumes" were not allowed to be higher than 6 inches above the knee, and men had to keep their chests covered while on the beach.

In 1925 Warner Brothers released the first talking picture show, "The Jazz Singer," starring Al Jolson, and a year later Ernest Hemingway published *The Sun Also Rises.* Robert Goddard launched the first liquid fuel rocket and, in 1927, transatlantic telephone service was established.

As for people in the news in 1927, Babe Ruth hit 60 home runs for the New York Yankees and Al Capone masterminded the St. Valentine's Day Massacre in Chicago. Admiral Richard Byrd had already made history by flying over the North Pole in his Fokker monoplane and was preparing to plant the American flag in Antarctica. Charles Lindbergh, in his Spirit of St. Louis, made the first nonstop flight from New York to Paris.

Internationally, Adolf Hitler was sentenced to five years imprisonment for attempting to overthrow the Bavarian government, but served less than one year, during which he wrote *Mein Kampf.* In Italy, Benito Mussolini — Il Duce — was coming to power and in Russia the Communist Congress expelled Leon Trotsky, bringing Joseph Stalin into power.

Within this historical context, the AART — and the x-ray industry — continued to make substantial headway as the decade of the '20s came to a close. During the Society's third annual meeting, Jerman reiterated his belief that for the organization to continue to grow, cooperation was paramount. Jerman said: "Be active in your local, state and national organizations; never be satisfied until the highest

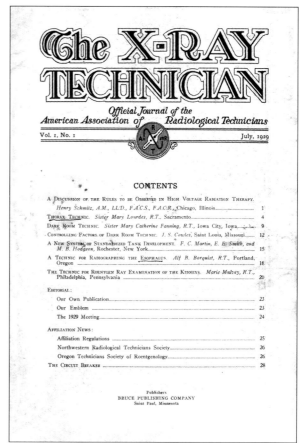

July 1929 – *The cover of the first issue of* The X-Ray Technician, *the official journal of AART.*

goals have been attained."

Practically every section of the country was represented at this meeting, and Jerman stressed the importance of the continuing development of local societies as affiliates of the AART. To this end, Jerman made a plea regarding "the value of more education and higher standards and the importance of national registration of x-ray technicians, not state registration."

The vision that Jerman pursued — the cementing of a viable national organization — still faced numerous obstacles. Linkage between the AART and the Registry, in Jerman's mind, may have been the strongest leverage available to convince those practicing radiologists who remained dubious that technicians' status as professionals was inevitable. During the AART's fourth annual meeting in 1929, it was obvious that others were beginning to share Jerman's vision. Fourteen new societies applied for affiliation.

Ed Jerman, now 64 years old, began to slowly turn the reins of the AART over to a younger generation. In 1929 Emma C. Grierson became president of the AART, and Margaret Hoing, Thomas Lough, Alfred B. Greene and H.A. Tuttle would become recognized as the new leaders of the organization. During this same year, Jerman was awarded the degree of Doctor of Science by the Board of Trustees of his alma mater, Franklin College, in recognition "of his outstanding achievements in the field of x-ray."

Having already been recognized by the Registry as a "Master Radiological Technician," Jerman also filled the educational textbook void with publication of his *Modern X-Ray Technic* in 1928. A compilation of Jerman's notes and observations from the previous 20 years, the work was immediately recognized as the most relevant publication of its kind in the field. It changed the method of making a radiographic exposure from the "guess and hunch" method to one of deliberate and accurate calculation, establishing for the first time the four qualities that constitute the radiograph: density, contrast, detail and distortion. Jerman's book remained a criteria of excellence far into the 1950s.

Perhaps the most noteworthy event to come from the 1929 meeting was a proposal by H.A. Tuttle for the AART to publish a journal. "Letters were read from technicians throughout the country requesting some plan be made whereby the papers and other material presented at the (annual) meeting might be made available to the members who could not attend."

It was clearly indicated by the membership that an association journal was not only wanted, it was necessary. A representative of the Bruce Publishing Company offered to publish four issues annually at a subscription rate of one dollar, a fee which the AART's executive committee voted to include in the memberships dues. *The X-Ray Technician* was born, and "none of those who advocated this important activity could foresee the tremendous value it would be to technicians and to the growth of the Society."

Two months later, in July 1929, the first issue of the journal was published.

But on Thursday, Oct. 24, 1929, history would deal a telling blow to the future of American business. The day is better known as Black Thursday, when 16 million shares of stock were dumped and Wall Street crashed. Within three days, stock averages fell 68 points. The Great Depression had begun in earnest.

The Catholic Connection

Catholic nuns dominated the field of radiologic technology during the first 40 years of ASRT history. They established hospitals and organized medical education programs throughout the Midwest and into Oklahoma and Texas.

Radiologic technology pioneers like Sr. Mary Alacoque Anger of St. Louis and Sr. Mary Beatrice Merrigan of Oklahoma City promoted technologist professionalism and education before it became fashionable. At St. Louis University, Sr. Mary Alacoque helped found the only four-year radiologic technology program in the nation in the late 1920s, while Sr. Mary Beatrice chartered the Oklahoma Society of X-ray Technicians and was the first recorded registered technician.

According to the Catholic Health Association, in 1929 nuns managed all 624 Catholic private and charity hospitals. The Sisters of St. Mary of the Third Order of St. Francis, now known as the Franciscan Sisters of Mary in St. Louis, established hospitals as early as 1902 and opened the first charity hospital for blacks run by a white Sisterhood in St. Louis in 1933. It was also one of the first Catholic hospitals to use x-ray equipment.

Sister Hilda Rita Bickus joined the Franciscan Sisters of Mary in 1946 as one of three black candidates. St. Mary's Infirmary was run by the sisters and had just started a program for black women to enter the order. Not only was Sr. Hilda one of the first blacks to become a nun in the health care field, she also received her bachelor of science degree in radiologic technology from St. Louis University. She was appointed supervisor of the radiology department and director of the radiologic technician program at St. Mary's. She established a two-year radiologic technician education program at St. Joseph's Hospital in St. Charles, Mo., and also taught radiologic technology at St. Louis University throughout her career.

She always showed a deep concern for

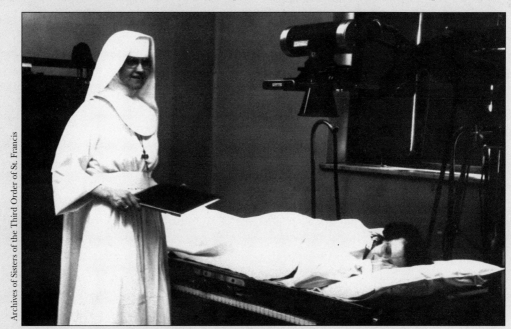

Archives of Sisters of the Third Order of St. Francis

Circa mid-1950s — X-ray room at St. Francis Hospital in Peoria, Ill.

the sick and the poor. One account of her childhood tells of her bringing home hungry children from other poor families. She also knew the suffering of the sick, having had her right leg amputated after an accident when she was 12. These experiences deepened her dedication to those in need and, like many nuns in health care, she was an inspiration to others. At her funeral in 1987 with her many friends and family, several of her former patients attended including one devoted person with an IV stand.

Members of the religious communities have been involved in the medical field since the Middle Ages. Most religious orders performed works of mercy serving at the first hospitals and ministering to the sick.

During the French Revolution, orders like the Daughters of Charity went into the neighborhoods to care for the sick. As medicine evolved, the nuns and religious orders adapted to meet the needs of the surrounding lay community.

The wave of Catholic Irish and German immigrants to the United States in the 1840s increased the need for Catholic hospitals and social programs. Immigrants often arrived in the country penniless, sick and unable to speak the language. Most hospitals and programs they encountered were Protestant, and although they met the physical and medical needs of this new population, the Protestant beliefs did not meet the immigrants' spiritual needs. It was common for hospitals to refuse a Catholic priest entrance to console and give last rites to a dying immigrant. Ostracized and seen as subjects of reform instead of charity by the Protestant community, immigrants didn't know where to turn until the Catholic religious responded by starting their own hospitals and social programs.

U.S. Catholic bishops asked the nuns to lead the way and establish hospitals and health education programs. Some orders had already entered health care because they saw a need. The Daughters of Charity took over the Baltimore Infirmary in 1823 and established other hospitals along the East Coast within five years. The Sisters of Mercy, the Third Order of St. Francis and the order of St. Joseph of Carondolet of St. Louis established a strong hospital network throughout the Midwest and into the western states. By 1871, 70 Catholic hospitals existed. In the next 25 years, more than 270 Catholic hospitals would meet the needs of the second wave of immigrants from Germany, Italy and Poland.

The Franciscan Sisters of St. Mary and the Congregation of Sisters of the Holy Family of Nazareth established orders in the United States to serve the special needs of German and Polish communities in St. Louis and Chicago. Other orders expanded service to the mining towns, lumber camps and railroad workers in the West.

Women wanting a professional career were sometimes better off becoming nuns. The opportunities and independence given nuns reached beyond accepted career boundaries for women in the first half of the 20th century. Sisters were given good opportunities because they were the only "qualified" appointees who could fulfill Catholic Church ministries.

"The Church appointed nuns out of solicitude to provide the best service. Sisters started as technicians, then department heads and moved to educational program development and eventually hospital administration," said Sister Stella Louise Slomka of the Congregation of Sisters of the Holy Family of Nazareth, a former radiologic technologist and chief executive officer of St. Mary of Nazareth Hospital Center in Chicago.

Many Sisters entered the radiologic technology profession during World War I when the majority of x-ray technicians, who were men, were conscripted. The Sisters adapted and learned to perform x-ray exams. Some of these nuns were registered nurses, while others had minimal health care training before going into x-ray.

According to Sr. Agnes Therese Duffy of the Order of St. Joseph of Orange in California, "Most of the x-ray training was taught on the job. Arthur Fuchs of General Electric gave some instruction to the nuns on how to use equipment, but technique was learned by watching the radiologist or through your own experience."

Other nuns worked a full day, then attended classes in the evenings to learn about nursing or radiologic technology. "We demanded it from ourselves to be well educated in order to give the best care to our patients," explains Sr. Stella Louise. ASRT archives show nuns comprised about 30 percent of the membership by the early 1930s.

The numbers of Catholic sponsored hospitals grew to 814 by 1961, but nuns held less visible roles as lay personnel became more involved in Catholic hospital operations and with the reforms of the Catholic church in the mid-1960s.

"One of the goals of the Sisters in our order was to captivate the lay people to carry on the mission and values of the hospital. I think the decrease in nuns in Catholic hospitals is due to the increase of good, strong lay substitutes in the Church's ministries," said Sr. Stella Louise.

Today, nuns sponsor more than 600 hospitals in the United States, and the majority sit on governing boards or as chief executive officers to see that the hospital's founding mission and values are maintained. The Catholic nuns established professional and educational standards for radiologic technology. Their dedication and leadership forever will be a vital part of the profession's history.

–Barbara Pongracz-Bartha

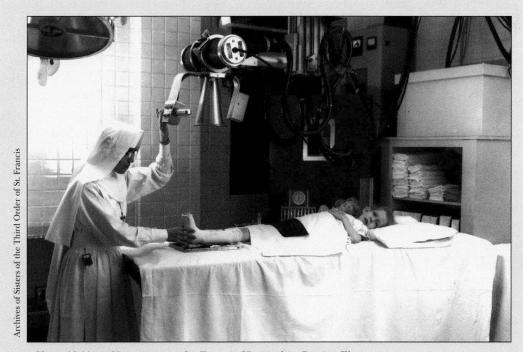

Archives of Sisters of the Third Order of St. Francis

Circa 1961 — X-ray room at St. Francis Hospital in Peoria, Ill.

Chapter Five

Setting the Standards

The widespread impact of the Great Depression did not bypass any segment of American enterprise, although the practice of medicine was spared the harshest effects of those economically difficult times. But as the Depression's influence filtered down through the ranks of business, the RSNA and ARRS eventually felt the inevitable pinch.

Funding for the Registry, which had no treasury of its own, was discontinued by the physicians, leaving the economic end of the operation to be run on a contingent basis. Renewal fees were charged to balance income with expenses. It was, however, a difficult proposition, and it delayed growth so necessary to the organization.

With the vast majority of Americans fighting for economic survival, the quest for technicians' professional status was replaced with the joy of simply having a job. Improving one's status was no longer a necessary priority. As soup lines became the common sight exemplifying the harshness of the times, many of the ordinary means by which technicians hoped to better themselves were not available. Advancing one's education was a luxury few could afford.

The AART appeared to be the only viable alternative to fill the educational void. Despite the country's horrendous difficulties, the fifth annual meeting of the Society took place, once again in Chicago. Although the attendance was modest — only 30 members and guests attended the first affiliation breakfast — 55 new members were accepted into the Society's ranks.

Two significant events occurred at this meeting. The first dealt with the confusion existing between the names of the AART and the ARRT. Because of this, the professional association's name was officially changed to the American Society of Radiographers (ASR). Additionally, the ASR was given the "privilege of representation" on the Registry Board. Professor Jerman, who had served as examiner for the previous six years, was asked to sit on the Registry Board to represent the Society. During the ASR meeting, Jerman also received the title of President Emeritus in recognition of his leadership.

In light of the economic woes, it is also interesting to note that the secretary-treasurer reported a balance of $1,113.60 in the Society's treasury. One year later, as a testament to frugal policies in hard times, the ASR's coffer had grown to $1,270.07. The sixth annual meeting of the ASR introduced a break with

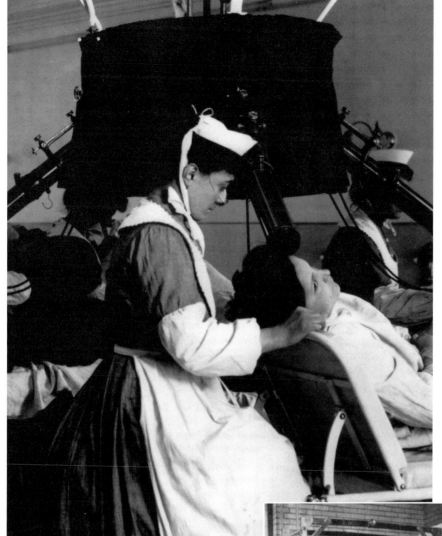

Art Resource Inc.

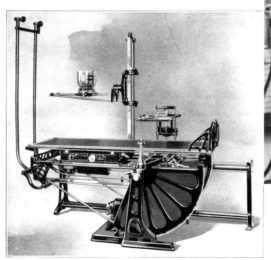

ASRT

Circa 1900 - *(left)*
The x-ray came into common use as a diagnostic tool.

Circa 1930 - *(below left)*
The Aurora x-ray table.

Circa 1936 - *(lower right)*
Mass x-rays were conducted to detect TB in the general population.

Reprinted with permission of the American Lung Association

the past, meeting in St. Paul, Minn., rather than Chicago. The 1931 meeting site was in response to member requests to schedule the conference in different areas of the country. By 1931 membership in the ASR had grown to 357 members.

In an effort to elevate the standards of radiographers and to raise the qualifications for registration, a Council on Education and Registration was created in cooperation with RSNA. The Council's chief function was to communicate with radiological organizations and hospitals to solicit their advice and support to establish "courses of study for radiographers" in educational institutions.

While the Council was not immediately successful with this, it was able to formally describe what technician training should include.

Modifications of this plan were adopted during the eighth annual meeting of the ASR in 1933.

Education and credibility for the technician's craft became synonymous — while remaining an acrimonious issue. What may have alarmed physicians most was the very

RSNA Council Recommendations - 1933

◆ All candidates should be 21 years of age and have "good health and personality as is required of candidates for admission in the First-Class Nurses Training Schools throughout the country."

◆ All courses in radiography should be given only in hospitals of at least 100-bed capacity and maintaining an accredited Nurses Training School, or in large medical clinics approved of by both the Council on Education and Registration and by the Board of the American Registry of X-Ray Technicians.

◆ The minimum time of the course should be for one full calendar year, and all students should devote their "entire time and energies to this course and not be expected nor permitted to do any other work during the entire year."

◆ The course of instruction must cover the following subjects:

1. General elementary anatomy and osteology, region and surface anatomy — 12 weeks
2. Physiology — 12 weeks
3. Nomenclature and terminology — Full year
4. Fundamentals of physics and electricity, including light and x-rays — 12 weeks
5. Roentgen apparatus and mechanics — 40 weeks
6. X-ray tubes and production of x-rays — 4 weeks
7. Darkroom chemistry and technic — 12 weeks
8. Basic technic factors and development of technic for all standardized procedures in radiography, and demonstration and practice of exposure technic for various parts of the body; rapid, slow, soft tissue work, etc., including effect of the factors of technic: kilovolts, milliamperes, distance, time — 40 weeks
9. Bedside unit: construction, operation and technic — 4 weeks
10. Electrical and radiation dangers and protection; troubleshooting — 40 weeks
11. Positioning — 40 weeks
12. Filing records; record keeping, history taking; typing — 12 weeks
13. Ethics; department management — 12 weeks
14. Calibration of machines — 4 weeks
15. Preparation of patient — 12 weeks
16. Technic of fluoroscopy — 4 weeks
17. Management of casts and splints — 12 weeks

necessity of what technicians did. Even with the spread of technician registration, certain radiologists voiced their concern that a registration certificate gave legitimacy, regardless of whether the technician practiced under a radiologist or chose an independent laboratory in which to work.

One of the hot points was the proscribed training necessary to become a technician. This eventually led the Registry to reevaluate its testing procedures. It found the examinations had become stereotyped. By 1927 five sets of examinations, consisting of five questions each, had been used for several years. Complete copies of all of the questions could be secured easily.

Further, no attempts were made to see whether or not the technician was living up to the agreement to uphold the professional "ethic" at the time of application, even though the consideration was quite straightforward:

> "If I receive a certificate from the American Registry of Radiological Technicians, I _____ hereby agree to work at all times under direct medical supervision, and under no circumstances to give out written or oral diagnoses or work independently, whether in any private office, hospital or institutional laboratory.
>
> (Signed)_____ "

Changes were obviously in order, and as Professor Jerman's health again began to fail, Alfred B. Greene was chosen as a liaison between the Registry and the ASR. Greene eventually was named executive secretary to the Registry Board in 1934. Jerman's health, however, was not the only reason for this move. The RSNA was still suspicious of commercial representatives attempting to gain a foothold in the ASR and RSNA. At the time, Jerman was still employed by the Victor Company, which had been purchased in 1920 by General Electric.

In the late 1920s, General Electric was embroiled in a controversy over its patent on the Coolidge cathode ray tube and its demands that the U.S. government impose prohibitive tariffs on the import of competing tubes from Europe. Members of the RSNA, upset that they could not obtain the less expensive European tubes, accused GE of holding a monopoly and eventually joined a lawsuit challenging its patent on the Coolidge tube. The animosity between the radiologists and General Electric cast an unfavorable light upon all GE employees, including Ed Jerman. Rumors began circulating that Jerman might be using his position as examiner for the Registry to the advantage of GE.

Although there may have been isolated cases of such problems with other individuals, for Jerman it was as untrue as it was unjust. But rather than risk harm to the ideals that he had worked so hard to establish, Jerman decided to "lessen the complications engendered by popular opinion" and resigned from the Registry in 1932. Fortunately, Greene proved to be as equally competent as Jerman.

As Greene later wrote in his *History of the Registry*, the Registry Board admitted that the organization was on the verge of "dry rot," and chose Greene because it was thought that "it might help to have the business management in the hands of someone closer to the technicians and their work." In short, Greene not only replaced Jerman, but was offered a salary by the Registry as well, hoping that "a participating incentive might be more effective."

What was unsaid during this change was that while the ASR enjoyed a comfortable budget surplus, the Registry had a reported loss of $500. Within a year, however, red ink had turned black. Whether it was Greene's business acumen that was responsible for this is unknown, but during his first year as execu-

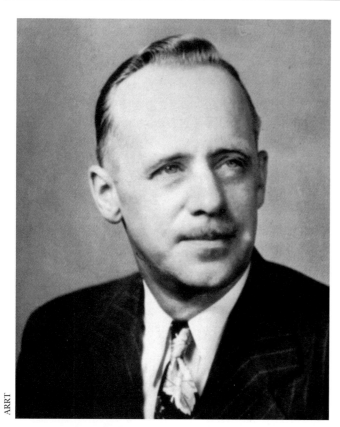

ARRT

1898 - 1982 – Alfred B. Greene

tive secretary, the Registry "gambled on their trust and reduced the application fee to $7 and the renewal charges to $1.50."

In truth, Greene assumed quite a role. As executive secretary, he was in charge of "preparing the various forms, organizing the clerical work, and attending to the business affairs of the Registry." During Greene's tenure, the organization changed its name from the American Registry of Radiological Technicians to the American Registry of X-Ray Technicians.

Dramatic changes also were made in examination practices as a result of recommendations coming from the Council on Education and Registration. Written verification procedures were instituted for those individuals listed as references for Registry applications. In most cases, radiologists sponsored technicians. Additionally, a high school education was

made a prerequisite for examination, with discretionary powers left to the Registry Board in accepting other preparation as being equivalent to high school, such as nurse training, night school courses, extension courses and college entrance examinations.

Place and manner of x-ray training and experience also were made considerations for application approval, with "time spent in various inadequate and commercially operated diploma mills discounted from the required training period." Additionally, a status of "associate" was established to designate technicians whose qualifications and examinations were approved by the Registry, but whose places of employment, "although ethical," were not under the supervision of a recognized radiologist. The term "associate" did not "lessen the degree of registration but defined, rather, the class of employee supervision."

The original five sets of questions were replaced with a master list of several hundred questions, thereby allowing different questions to be selected for different groups of applicants. The new examinations consisted of 10 groups of three questions each. The applicant was given a choice of two questions out of each three, making a total of 20 questions to be answered. The passing grade for the examination also was raised to 75 percent.

A final group of three questions was added dealing with "professional ethics." When this was instituted, according to Greene, "many applicants were rejected for failure to make proper replies to the ethical questions; but it soon became apparent that no technician properly schooled in ethics would deliberately condemn himself in an examination; and the information acquired in the ethical section... could be used to correct an improper situation and instruct the technician properly along these lines." So the grade on ethics was separated from the other grades and considered separately, and a technician often passed without reexamination "when his misunderstandings had been cleared up."

This business of ethics was taken seriously, and as Greene streamlined both paperwork and procedures, the Registry began to assert more control over these ethical questions, developing the methodology to keep track of the growing number of registered technicians. Renewal of registration not only involved paying dues, but a "signed attest and renewal agreement testifying to the applicant's adherence to ethical tenets."

For technicians not employed or engaged in other x-ray work — the use of x-ray in industrial applications was becoming increasingly common — a special form was provided giving the Registry data on which to decide whether a technician should be carried in good standing. For those accepted for renewal a dated seal and registration card were provided, designating whether the technician was "regular" or "associate."

Greene wrote, "The good faith of the Registry in abiding by these standards was shown when a technician, prominent in technician affairs, was dropped from the Registry, and subsequently from the ASR, after establishing an independently operated laboratory." Steps were also taken to see that "proper publicity" concerning the Registry appear in radiologic journals, including *The X-Ray Technician.*

As the Registry raised itself from the doldrums, the ASR continued to grow in size and strength. In 1932 changes in the bylaws again were made dealing with the name of the organization. The American Society of Radiographers officially became the American Society of X-Ray Technicians (ASXT) during the 1934 annual meeting, the last name change until 1964, when the Society adopted its present designation, ASRT — the American Society of Radiologic Technologists.

The Depression wore on, tightening its grip. Effects were finally felt within the Reg-

istry, with Alfred Greene voluntarily reducing his own salary by 50 percent "in order to keep the Registry financially sound." His pay was reinstated the following year, as Greene accepted other responsibilities. Due to the untimely death of Emma Grierson in 1932, Greene assumed additional responsibilities as editor of *The X-Ray Technician.*

In 1935 the ASXT broke with Upper Midwest tradition and held its 10th annual meeting in Dallas, but the meeting venue reflected the times. For the first time the Society recorded its definite opposition to "the unionistic activities of some technicians and hospital workers in some parts of the country." The following resolution was adopted:

> Be It Resolved: That The American Society of X-Ray Technicians go on record as being opposed to "strikes and lockouts" as a method of settling financial differences, in hospitals and medical clinics, where care of the sick and afflicted may in any way be impaired. The object of this Society is educational, "to promote the Science and the Art of Radiography" and as trained technicians to give the highest type of service to mankind in efficient aid to the medical profession. As a Society we have no sympathy with collective bargaining or other forms of unionism.

There is no doubt that the ASXT was in strong hands, persevering in its quest toward the legitimate recognition of technicians. That it oftentimes mirrored the possible paranoia of the Registry, and therefore the RSNA, was a sign of the times. But it was necessary. Seeking control over its own fate and the fate of its members was paramount. Maintaining the strength of the Society, both in terms of its financial stability and membership, had given rise to a certain amount of political clout.

This was manifested in 1936, when the ASXT was authorized to make two appointments to the Registry Board. The first two members to serve in this capacity were Thomas Lough, R.T., and Roy E. Wolcott, R.T. Although the Registry Board now consisted of four radiologists and two technicians, the progression toward eventual self management of technicians' destiny had begun.

Professor Jerman's dream was becoming reality.

There can be no doubt that Professor Jerman was dedicated to his vision, but with advancing age, an ongoing battle with arteriosclerosis and the cumulative effect of years of exposure to x-rays, he apparently withdrew from active participation in the various organizations. This did not mean Jerman completely disappeared. During the late '20s and early '30s, Jerman and his daughter traveled extensively, revisiting England, Europe, South America and Cuba. In each country he stopped to discuss x-ray techniques with leaders in the field.

But who was Jerman, the man, to have withdrawn so completely from the limelight on his home turf? Sister Mary Beatrice Merrigan, Jerman's close friend, described him as being "small in stature, and apparently quite frail; his eyes were most expressive — blue and very bright. A slight lisp in speech accounted for his greater effort to enunciate clearly when teaching. His hair became iron-gray in his later years. He possessed a quiet manner and appeared a bit timid."

Dr. Edward H. Skinner remarked of Jerman: "He was neat, and always showed good taste in dress, and wore well-fitting clothes. He was ever apparently of the same height and appearance. I believe I never knew anyone else who kept the same stature and appearance throughout a matter of thirty-five years. About the only feature that changed was the gradual graying of his hair, and even

that was hardly noticeable."

Sister Mary Beatrice noted: "Professor Jerman was to everyone he met, a kindly, friendly and benign person, never imposing his personality upon anyone, and never forcing his salesmanship ability. He practically let a prospective purchaser sell himself. He had a shrewd, kindly sense of humor, and was never at a loss for a pleasant story to tell. The following one he insisted is true: One hot summer day he was walking downtown and came to a small group of youngsters selling lemonade. The price was two glasses for a nickel. He bought and drank two glasses, then continued his walk. A block or two further he met some other young lemonade merchants, who said their price was a nickel for one glass. When Jerman asked for the reason of the difference in price, the second merchants answered: 'Their puppy fell into their lemonade'."

Jerman's various biographers attest to his frail condition. Sister Mary Beatrice wrote, "He was never very strong physically, but he had a tremendous amount of energy. He ate little, but was very definite as to what that little should be. For breakfast he chose a cup of coffee and a glass of milk and into the milk always broke a piece of bread. Most waitresses could not understand his ordering both milk and coffee, and would serve him only one; on such occasions they saw a flare of temper rarely known to his associates.

"Professor Jerman loved company and therefore found life very lonely away from home. He particularly disliked being alone in the evening, and invariably worked in his classroom, experimenting or studying on those occasions. He often told the students of his ambitions for the department, and of the grand opportunities it offered. His students greatly profited by his loneliness."

Jerman's personal side was no less peculiar or deliberate. According to Sister Mary Beatrice, "(He) was a great lover of music, and

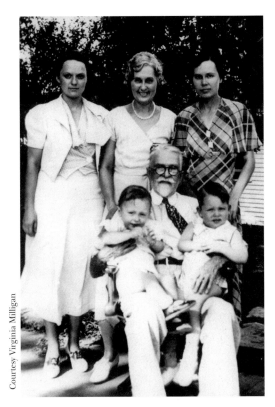

Courtesy Virginia Milligan

Circa 1934 - *Ed C. Jerman with his family. Jerman died September 13, 1936.*

although he had not been trained to sing or play an instrument, he bought one of the first phonographs made. He owned more than five hundred records — and enjoyed only classical and semi-classical selection. During his years of travel he acquired many records typical of the countries he visited. He states that he owned the first piano and the first cylindrical phonograph in Indiana, and told his grand-daughters that he would buy them any musical instrument on condition that they would learn to play it."

Jerman obviously inherited much from his parents, for Sister Mary Beatrice described him as a man "who loved children, and he took his grandchildren to all the National Parks in the West. He strove to instill the virtue of thrift into these little girls, and one year he promised, as a Christmas gift, to match the greatest amount they could save.

(He) was anxious to train his grand-children in a spirit of honesty, and when one of them came home from school crying because she had been accused of saying something that was not true, the grandfather asked the child: 'Are you sure you didn't say it?' 'Yes, I'm sure,' said the little girl. 'Well,' said Jerman, 'You then have nothing about which you need to feel sorry.'"

Jerman, the researcher, had always impressed his colleagues. He undertook a number of studies, notable among them being the radiography of Egyptian and Peruvian mummies at the Field Museum in Chicago, where x-ray equipment was installed and thousands of radiographs made for a pathologic study.

After his retirement, Jerman continued to work assiduously at his various hobbies and interests at home. He was a great reader of biology, botany and genealogy. H.O. Mahoney, Jerman's colleague at General Electric, said he never had known anyone of the same patience, vision and determination. In all his teachings and lecturing Jerman insisted most strongly upon carrying out the details necessary to obtain good technical results. Once, when asked how he succeeded in developing x-ray techniques, Jerman told the story of the Englishman who invented the needle of the shoelace. Someone had asked the latter how he happened to think of it, and he replied: "By not thinking of anything else for twenty years."

Perhaps most indicative of Jerman was his concern for the patients with whom he came into contact. When involved in taking x-rays, Jerman often said to them: "Put the hurt on the film."

His own pain, however, caught up with him quickly after his retirement. On Sept. 4, 1935, Jerman wrote a letter to ASXT historian Margaret Hoing in response to a scrapbook she had sent. His letter read:

New Rules for Protection in the '40s

During the early days of the profession, radiation protection for the patient and the technician wasn't strictly enforced. Many pioneers suffered greatly from the effects of overexposure to radiation. As late as the 1930s, pregnant women were x-rayed to determine the health of their baby, and technicians had to hold patients during exams.

In September 1940, the U.S. National Bureau of Standards helped establish the daily maximum amount of radiation for individuals — 1/10th of an r-unit per day, with anything in excess considered to be a hazard to the worker. The Bureau suggested that technicians refuse to hold uncooperative patients during x-rays, and that x-ray departments should have an "inviolate" rule to this effect to avoid unnecessary direct radiation.

The Bureau of Standards also published data regarding the thickness of lead required to stop radiation of varying voltages. "The 'hardness' or penetrating power of x-rays increases with a rise in voltage, so lead thickness should increase proportionally — for example, if roentgen rays generated by peak voltages do not exceed 250 kV, then the minimum equivalent thickness of lead is 6.00 mm."

A study was conducted of the personnel of a large radiology laboratory at a general hospital and found that the number of red blood cells were slightly increased more often than they were decreased in persons with chronic exposure. There was also a slight increase in hemoglobin concentration. The study noted that large doses of radiation produced the opposite effect — anemia.

Scattered radiation was also now of concern. It was found that 0.0005 r/milliampere second was scattered from a patient during fluoroscopic examination on a contemporary fluoroscopic table. "The safe time for the technician to stand within ten inches of the patient was 200 microseconds or forty seconds when a large field is employed." Fortunately, the size of the field was generally small. However, the technicians were told to "keep as far as possible from the x-ray beam" and to "always use the recommended thickness of lead."

Protection for the x-ray technician was greatly improved as a result of these and other scientific studies during and after the war. A study done in 1940 determined that out of 91 x-ray workers, 24.2 percent were sterile. The dangers of radiation had become apparent, and as a result, it was recommended that:

1. Photofluorographic units be housed in rooms of at least 18 by 12 feet.
2. X-ray machines be at least 8 to 10 feet from the side walls to reduce reflected radiation.
3. X-ray tubes be properly aligned to prevent stray radiation.
4. Scatter radiation from tube leakage be reduced by confining the primary beam to the area of the screen.
5. Protective screens with lead shielding of 0.1 to 0.2 mm thickness be used.
6. Operators be required to stand behind screens during all exposures.
7. Exposure be determined by using a wire mesh.
8. Occupational radiation exposure be measured by dental films worn by technicians for seven day periods.
9. Routine blood counts of technicians be made each month.

Other suggestions indicated safety concerns persisted, though scientific answers were not exactly up to the task. Black x-ray technicians, for instance, were considered less threatened by excess radiation because of the pigment in their skin. Other ideas even less scientifically sound were observed.

Radiation was not the only concern, of course. Darkrooms were frequently quite cramped with no ventilation, and it was not uncommon for technicians to mix their own developing and fixing chemicals.

— *Barbara Pongracz-Bartha*

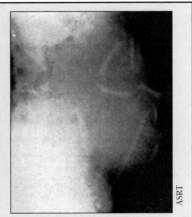

Circa 1931 - *A lateral view of a full term pregnancy.*

Dear Miss Hoing:

I want to thank you for the beautiful scrapbook you made and sent to me. It was a nice piece of work. I am sure all will appreciate it. I had my fifth surgical operation two weeks ago. Removal of the x-ray growths from my left arm. It is slow in healing but looks as though it would heal all right eventually. It began to show some signs of malignancy and proved to be epithelioma in the early stages. My greatest trouble now is a faulty circulation which prevents me from walking much although I can get around in the car frequently. I expect to go to California for a week or two maybe a month soon. My regards to Dr. Orndorff, yourself and other friends.

With Kindest Regards,
Ed C. Jerman

Within a short time, Jerman's circulatory problems worsened. One leg was eventually amputated. "During his last days he remained constantly in bed, but was patient and cheerful, retaining his spirit of humor to the last."

He died Sept. 13, 1936.

An appropriate obituary was noted in both *The X-Ray Technician* and in the October 1936 edition of the *Victor News*, a newsletter published by General Electric. However, no formal mention of Jerman's death was addressed at the 1937 meeting of the ASXT.

Tributes to Jerman would come later, penned by his lifelong friend, Margaret Hoing, R.T. "Professor Ed C. Jerman was our direct link with Roentgen's discovery," Hoing wrote in 1948. Four years later she dedicated her *History of the ASXT* to the professor, writing, "Far beyond the feeling of gratitude to him for his life of usefulness to humanity, through which he — more than any other one in his day — carried advanced technical radiology to the other countries of the world, there remains in the heart of all of those who knew him personally an admiration and love for him as a gentleman, and a friend, and as a teacher."

Former ASXT President Thomas Lough, R.T., expressed similar sentiments in 1952. Lough wrote:

"My mind travels along memory's trail to the first meeting with Ed C. Jerman and the impressions of that day at the Province Hospital in Seattle in 1921. It was the beginning of a series of class studies of x-ray technique, and I was to attend the evening sessions. At this time he told the story of the 'hunch' method and the 'scientific' method, later published in the introductory chapter of *Modern X-Ray Technic.*

"Upon the wall of my office in the Swedish Hospital hangs a photographic likeness of Professor Jerman, which bears the legend I placed there: 'The world's greatest technician.' It was felt that he had done more to standardize technique than any other man. Among my most highly prized books is a leather-bound copy of *Modern X-Ray Technic* in which is written, With the compliments of the author, Ed C. Jerman.

"The call came early in 1936 which placed him among the martyrs of science from Roentgen rays."

Jerman's legacy, far more powerful than his death, continued to exert influences on the future of x-ray technicians and the Society he founded. Uppermost in the collective mind of the ASXT throughout the late 1930s was the question of ethics. The rumored influence of unionism could not be quelled. In 1939 during the 13th annual meeting held in Madison, Wis., the ASXT again voiced its opposition to the idea. For years, the prevailing though unstated attitude of radiologists at large had been one of skepticism regarding the eventual aims of x-ray technicians in building a large and influential national organization. Aware of their own uncertain situation in medical economics, the radiologists watched technicians for trends that might lead to concerted demands that the physicians might not be able to fulfill.

While the attitude of the technicians "had been tacitly understood among themselves, there had been... no attempt to crystallize this sentiment" to be adopted as a Society policy. The desire to avoid antagonism with other organizations had kept them "somewhat in a passive attitude." But the growing sense of uncertainty among technicians made it more expedient for the Society to adopt a definite code, which took the form of a lengthy resolution, ending:

"THEREFORE, BE IT RESOLVED that the American Society of X-Ray Technicians does hereby declare that the affiliation of our members with trade unions or other similar organizations is incompatible with the obligation of professional men and women and hence detrimental to public welfare."

The issue of unionism, hopefully, was laid to rest. The question of ethics, at least in the mind of the radiologist, was assuaged. The ASXT, after 20 years of striving for professional credibility, had reached a new beginning, a new plateau, from which technicians could at last find themselves a rank of stature in the medical community.

In addition, the profession had to deal with unresolved safety issues. With many pioneers of roentgenology suffering from the effects of overexposure to x-rays, safety standards crept back into the collective consciousness. During the 1930s radiologists, technicians and manufacturers began to experiment with preventative measures.

In 1937 the International X-Ray and Radium Protection Commission issued new safety guidelines for full-time x-ray workers: not more than seven working hours per day; not more than five working days per week — and days off were to be spent outdoors; not less than one month's vacation per year; and no extra shifts for other hospital duties.

How closely these guidelines were followed is unclear. Some institutions even decades later encouraged technicians to eat at least one meal of cooked liver per week to cleanse the system. Many technicians remained unaware of preventative measures good or bad, especially those self-taught and in small towns. The value of safety training was paramount for the physician societies and the ARXT, although specific precautions varied little throughout the '30s and '40s.

From manufacturers' points of view, devel-

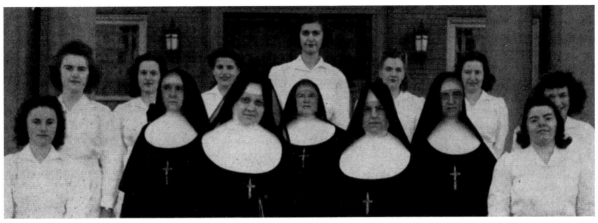

Circa 1942 – Students in the radiologic technology program at the St. Louis University School of Nursing.

oping safer tubes and mechanisms was in their best interest. Shielded tubes introduced during this period prevented radiation leakage, and electrical hazards from ungrounded equipment were eliminated. The Keleket X-Ray Corporation continued to introduce safer techniques, having fully developed a penetration per part technique to help standardize x-ray technology. Two times the thickness of a patient plus the constant 27 gave the minimum kVp needed for adequate penetration of a specific body part. Based on this technique, Keleket's equipment was widely accepted, although some members of the profession berated the inventors of the unit for making it possible for anyone to take x-ray pictures.

Advancements in film also made the technician's job easier. In 1933 an acetate safety base film was introduced, replacing the dangerous nitrate-based film. In 1931 Frank Thomas Powers was the first to make radiographic paper on rolls with which two chest radiographs per minute could be taken at a cost of about 75¢ each, and in 1936 Ansco introduced a non-screen x-ray film for direct exposure techniques.

It had been a turbulent 10 years for technicians and America. The effects of the American Depression were felt worldwide, with few countries remaining economically unscathed. As a result of this, the United States followed Great Britain in dropping its currency from the gold standard in 1933. In other international events, the Chinese Civil War began, introducing the names Mao Tse-tung and Chaing Kai-shek to the general press.

In the United States, diversion from the Depression led to what some considered the greatest radio hoax of all times — Orson Welles' broadcast of "*The War of the Worlds.*" In Hollywood, Walt Disney Studios began work on the first full-length animated feature, "*Snow White and the Seven Dwarfs,*" and "*Gone With the Wind*" began production.

Having survived the worst of times relatively unscathed, the ranks of the ASXT's registered technicians, now more than 1,100 strong, soon faced yet another adversary. By 1936 American joblessness reached 10 million as a result of the Depression, but Franklin Roosevelt's New Deal brought a ray of hope. Then on July 19, 1936, the Spanish Civil War began, bringing Franco into power, and on Sept. 1, 1939, Adolf Hitler's armies invaded Poland. The world was again at war.

Combatting the 'Great White Plague'

In one of the nation's longest and most comprehensive public health battles, the U.S. government during the 1930s and '40s launched a ferocious attack against "the great white plague" — tuberculosis. Known throughout the world for centuries as "consumption," the easily-spread bacterial infection first reached epidemic proportions in the United States in the early 1900s. By the 1940s, tuberculosis was responsible for more deaths in the United States than any other contagious disease.

Because tuberculosis is symptom-free in its early stages, one of the few ways to detect the disease in the 1940s was through an x-ray of the chest. The U.S. Public Health Service responded with an intense control effort involving mass tuberculosis screenings, where patients were x-rayed in assembly-line fashion in factories, school gymnasiums and clinics. These screenings, conducted in urban areas coast to coast, involved millions of dollars of radiographic equipment.

X-ray technicians played a vital role in the tuberculosis screenings of the era. One of the nation's largest TB surveys, designated as "Operation-TB," was conducted in Cuyahoga County, Ohio, from March 9 to Aug. 20, 1949. The Public Health Service's Division of Tuberculosis Control installed 25 portable and mobile x-ray units in area factories, schools and stores in an effort to x-ray everyone in the county older than 15. During the five-month period, free screenings were performed on 684,763 people. Those whose radiographs showed abnormalities were notified, by mail, to report to a retake center where detailed medical histories were obtained and another chest x-ray was taken. During the height of Operation-TB, each x-ray technician performed hundreds of exams a day and as many as 40 rolls of 100-foot-long x-ray film were processed daily.

In other mass TB screenings during the late 1940s, more than 300,000 people were x-rayed in the Denver area; 454,130 were examined in Washington, D.C.; and 536,014 were screened in Boston. The largest x-ray

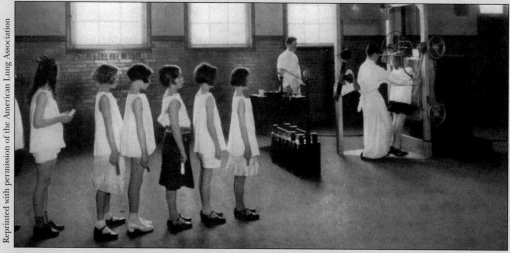

Reprinted with permission of the American Lung Association

Circa 1931 - Mass chest x-rays begin in a Long Island public school in a search for TB.

survey in U.S. history, however, began in Los Angeles on March 22, 1950. Technicians using 40 mobile x-ray units screened their one-millionth person on Sept. 14, 1950, and by the time the program ended on Dec. 31 of that year, 1.7 million people throughout Los Angeles County had been screened and thousands of cases of TB had been detected. Each technician involved in the effort was making between 1,500 and 2,000 exposures a week.

These mass screenings created a nationwide demand for trained x-ray technicians who could produce uniform diagnostic x-rays of the chest. Many urban areas reported shortages of qualified x-ray technicians, leading to active recruitment by the profession and rapid growth in the number of x-ray schools and programs. Between 1940 and 1946, the number of accredited schools for x-ray technicians increased by 45 percent.

But technical expertise wasn't the only demand on x-ray technicians performing mass radiography. Working out of school gymnasiums and public auditoriums, these technicians also had to be able to set up impromptu dressing rooms or turn storage closets into makeshift darkrooms. They serviced their own equipment and became adept at troubleshooting. And while screening workers at industrial plants, the x-ray technicians were responsible for maintaining a smooth schedule so the factory's production line wasn't interrupted.

The mass x-ray screenings — combined with the development of effective antibiotics, the sanatorium movement and better living conditions — helped reduce the death rate from tuberculosis in the United States from 43.4 per 100,000 people in 1944 to 4.1 per 100,000 people by 1967.

—Ceela McElveny

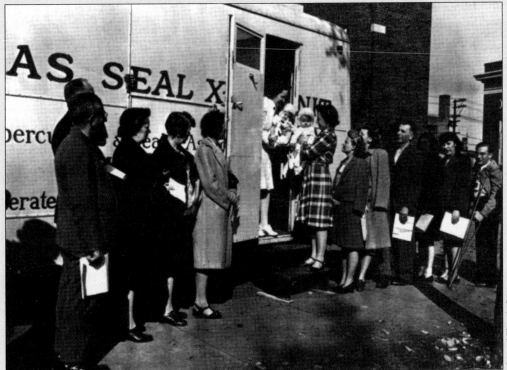

Circa 1950 - *Minnesota residents line up for TB screening at a mobile chest unit.*

General Electric Company

Chapter Six

The Images of War

The United States entered World War II in 1941, and as the conflict escalated, the value of every physically sound man and woman was of importance, whether they served in combat or on the home front.

The United States began mobilizing its medical forces before entering the war. The Army realized the important role roentgenologists and x-ray technicians had played in the previous war. The Army Medical School presented weekly lectures and presentations on radiology, and prepared a two-week crash course on the duties of a radiologist stationed at an induction station. But the Surgeon General realized that the numbers of radiologists being trained, plus those who volunteered, would hardly meet the expected demand in the field.

At the 12th annual conference of the American College of Radiology, Lt. Col. Alfred A. de Lorimer, MC, Commandant of the Army School of Roentgenology in World War II, described the situation: The Army needed roentgenologists who could assume duties of a general physician, making general diagnoses on large numbers of casualties in minimum time. X-ray and fluoroscopic viewing would be used more than in World War I

to diagnose injuries of the abdomen, chest and skull. Radiologists were in high demand but were a small group compared to other medical specialists; therefore, others would need to be trained in radiology fundamentals to meet the demand.

Roentgenologists and x-ray technicians served in a variety of situations. The field (surgical) hospital was the closest radiologic unit to the frontline. Surgeons treated non-transportable casualties and could perform as many as 80 surgeries in 24 hours. Two roentgenologists and three enlisted x-ray technicians manned the radiology department, performing fluoroscopy mostly, often in a tent or the back of a closed truck.

The evacuation hospital, approximately 30 to 70 miles behind the frontline, housed about 750 casualties with two roentgenologists and 10 technicians. Radiologists used both fluoroscopy and x-ray and still operated the darkroom out of tents. The doctors and technicians in field and evacuation hospitals had to "be self-reliant and resourceful and prepared to render quick judgements." Patients were sent on to general convalescent hospitals where three radiologists and nine technicians were allotted per 1,000 patients.

Initially the Army had two training pro-

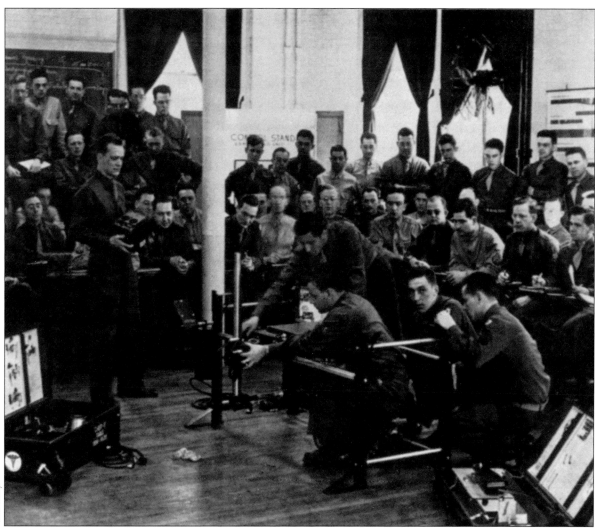

U.S. Army

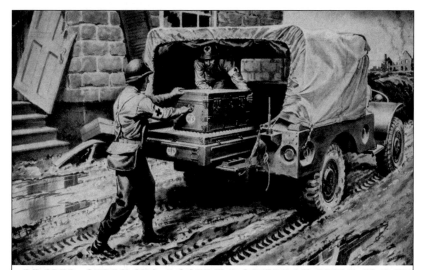

ASRT

ARMED SERVICES ACCEPT PORTABLE FIELD X-RAY
New Picker Unit Operates Anywhere: Assembles in 5 Minutes

1942 - (top)
*The November 1942 class of the
Army School of Roentgenology
assembling x-ray field equipment as
part of their final exam.*

1952 - (left)
Picker ad in The X-Ray Technician.

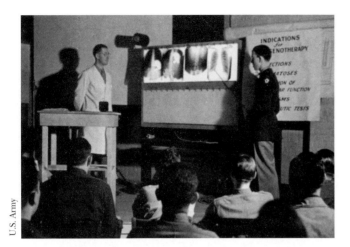

U.S. Army

Circa 1942 - *A seminar in diagnostic roentgenology being conducted by Lt. Col. Henry G. Moehring, MC, Chief, Clinical Section, Diagnostic Radiology.*

grams for radiologists. The shorter course was two weeks long and focused on exams conducted at induction centers. The longer course consisted of four weeks of emergency training, eight hours a day, six days a week of lectures, exams and conferences. Positioning was left to be learned in the field. Civilian radiologists criticized this training program and called its graduates "de Lorimer's 8-week wonders."

The war exerted subtle influences on technicians and would-be technicians across the United States. Appeals went out for registered technicians to enroll in emergency services established by the Red Cross and Army Medical Corps. These groups desperately wanted to establish a nucleus of x-ray technicians to be available in time of national emergency to act where and when they would most be needed. The call for x-ray technicians worked, with the number of registered technicians in the Armed Forces growing from 12 in 1942 to 131 in 1945.

The warning cries from the home front were immediate. Technicians were cautioned about abandoning their jobs to accept openings in government hospitals — "because of patriotic reasons, or for reaching out for bet-

ter remuneration." Rumors ran rampant. One such rumor particularly disturbing to the medical community was that the government was setting up a "vast" training program for Army technicians in order to replace civilian technicians. Military medical x-ray technicians could earn between $1,620 and $2,000 a year, and junior laboratory helpers could earn $1,440 a year.

Technicians responding to the call often chose the Red Cross. Much to the chagrin of the Registry, many of these technicians were rejected because of a lack of training under a recognized radiologist, or lack of a high school degree. Those technicians who did qualify were assigned a specialist's rating after completing basic training. Registered technicians serving in the Navy were also able to secure special rating, receiving the rank of Pharmacist's Mate 1st Class upon promotion. Rank upon enlistment was one grade higher for registered technicians than for unregistered technicians.

In reality, only a few hundred registered technicians responded with applications, and with an increasing number of those unable to qualify, the Army laid the rumors to rest and established a 90-day technician training program along with a quota in 16 Army training centers around the country. Each student was required to assemble and disassemble an x-ray unit to pass the final exam. The Army School of Roentgenology at the University of Tennessee graduated more than 1,400 technicians.

The Registry and ASXT responded carefully. A 1944 article in *The X-Ray Technician* stated, "Careful investigation of certain Army Training Schools for technicians resulted in special credit being given towards the requirement for registration to men completing these courses and following them with a required amount of satisfactory practical experience.

"Much of the training was given with the requirements of registration in mind; and technicians with sufficient experience and other qualifications were encouraged to register by their radiological superiors... There is no relaxation of standards in qualifying applicants in Service for registration, as it has been kept in mind that when these technicians return to civilian life, they will work and compete with the rank and file of the other registered technicians.

"In many cases it has been forethought on the part of the applicant which prompted him to secure proper recognition while still in the Army or Navy so that he would be definitely classified in case there was any question as to the extent and amount of his training later on."

What did this mean? In short, the Registry and ASXT suddenly found a prophetic voice regarding the problems they had long espoused about educational standards, or lack thereof. True, many of the registered technicians — perhaps those who were certified during the early years of the Registry — could not qualify as military technicians, but the Registry and ASXT recognized that legitimate training, whether in a college or in the service, could not harm their ultimate goals for upgrading educational prerequisites.

The war effort, through military training, provided what the AMA had refused in 1940. In 1940 the ASXT's Council on Education and Registration issued a plan for securing certain rights and protection for x-ray technicians. The plan called for increased publicity for the Registry to secure more cooperation from radiologists; recognition by the AMA or some other medical group of Registry-approved education courses; and some method whereby educational courses could be standardized and monitored.

The council also sought endorsement of a program to provide retirement or Social Security protection for x-ray technicians. At the time, x-ray technicians were unable to gain Social Security and unemployment benefits

The 90-Day Wonders

Starting in 1939, students accepted into Army radiography training came from every location possible. The fears expressed by the ASXT regarding qualifications were not without merit. Men with no more than grammar school background sometimes enrolled in classes covering mathematics, physics and chemistry for which "even though the instruction was elementary, they were totally unfit. And there were those students who, regardless of qualifications, lacked interest since they had no choice in their being assigned to train as Army radiographers."

By 1943 the training had been expanded to 120 days, and the Army had established the Army School of Roentgenology in Tennessee, where additional emphasis was placed on research projects "designed to solve such problems as breakages from inadequate packing methods, use of suspension cradles for under-table skull radiography, and determining uniform film identification strategies."

The training equipment was moved to Fort Sam Houston, in Texas, after the end of the war, where the only formal Army radiography training program remains today.

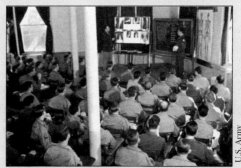

Circa 1942 - A class of Army Roentgenology students.

because they were employed in hospitals, clinics or institutions (religious, charitable, scientific, literary and educational), all of which were exempt from these federal programs.

The plan met with predictable results. The AMA refused to consider a lowering of training prerequisites, and radiologists could not agree on higher ones. The retirement and Social Security initiatives required a mandate of Congress, which did not seem immediately forthcoming.

By November 1942, the crunch in manpower caused by the war was of concern. The ASXT said, "The present world crisis has created a hitherto unthought of demand for x-ray technicians and as is the case in nearly every other field, the supply is far below the demand."

The daily press began carrying articles of so-called "raids" on x-ray personnel of one plant or factory by another manufacturer. A rosy picture of improved working conditions together with a promised increase in salary enticed employees away from a job. The situation was so desperate in some branches of industry as to affect war production, resulting in the government passing legislation to prevent workers from changing jobs.

The ASXT noted that "not all these raids are confined to war production industries, but (in) institutional and private x-ray departments. A great difference lies in the point that... these raids on x-ray technical personnel have been directed not at trained workers, but rather at student technicians."

At the same time, women technicians were asking how they could serve the war effort. Women were barred from the front lines. The ASXT noted that "it falls to the women to fill the gaps in the home ranks left vacant by the enlistment or drafting of many male technicians. While not as spectacular as service in uniform, it is as necessary as the retention of many other key people needed to maintain the care

Women's Work

During the war years, women's rights had not defined itself as a cohesive movement. In 1943 the female technician was usually in a private office, and was expected to do everything from operate the x-ray equipment to keep books and type correspondence. Although this "Jill of all trades" was exhorted to have common sense with regard to her duties, she was also expected to be neat, clean, unblemished, and "have no amputations that might startle or disgust the patient. Her uniform should always be fresh, her hair neat, her nails well kept and a minimum of cosmetics displayed. Her breath should be free from halitosis and her body free from body odors." Being courteous, tactful and sympathetic were also musts.

As for the requirements for male technicians, "sound health, poise and sureness and the ease with which he labors make a great impression on the patient. Any kind of personal uncleanliness makes the technician unacceptable to the patient, lessens his influence and mars his usefulness. A fresh, clean uniform, shoes polished, hair well groomed, no body odor and not too much of the present-day cosmetics . . ." were proscribed for men.

The Registry and ASXT promulgated such beliefs and practices. "Inquiries are not infrequently received by the Registry board as to the relative opportunities in the field of x-ray technique for men and women. At the present time both... are serving well... although there are certain circumstances and phases of work for which either one may be respectively better adapted. In a physician's office it is apparent that a woman is, in most cases, better able to act as a physician's assistant, or a receptionist, than a man. On the other hand, a woman would find certain types of industrial x-ray certainly out of her field.

"Many radiologists insist that the graduate nurse becomes the best technician because of her understanding of patient problems and medical procedures gained through her nursing education. Her adaptability to institutional routine and discipline is also likely to be greater. However, most men have a better understanding of the theoretical, electrical and mechanical aspects that pertain to the maintenance and operation of x-ray equipment and in institutions where such responsibilities can be entrusted to the technician, it has been found to be desirable (to have a male technician). Men are often able to undergo, better than women, the physical effort that busy departments require, although neither of the above is always the case.

"With proper training men can become as well fitted to understand and handle patients as women; in fact, there is an appreciable number of x-ray technicians who are graduate male nurses. Larger institutions are becoming more and more in favor of a male technician as head of the department with both sexes included in the assisting personnel. It is felt by some that a man can maintain a more impersonal discipline in a mixed group."

Sexual bias against women existed despite statistics showing only 20 percent of registered technicians were male in 1941.

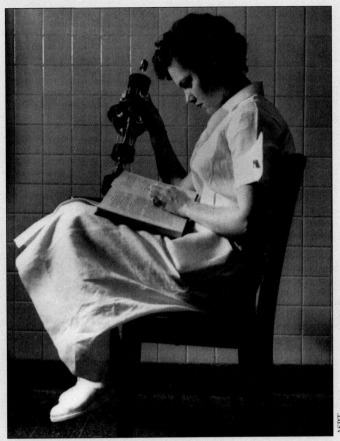

Circa 1945 – *A radiographer-in-training studies the properties of the x-ray tube to prepare for her Registry exam.*

The perception at the time was that "as a rule, male technicians remain longer in their positions and have less tendency to change than do women. Many of them have families and look to their positions as their living security; while a large number of girls entering the x-ray field do so with a feeling that it is temporary until marriage intervenes." The ASXT noted that despite the low percentage, the number of male applicants was growing.

The Registry and ASXT didn't favor either sex as being superior, "...since there is a field for both, the success of each individual depend(s) on his or her ability, adaptability and application."

of the civilian population. X-ray technicians who are graduate nurses have been urged to enlist as nurses, since the need for nurses is even greater than the need for technicians."

Thus, the female x-ray technicians who were left stateside virtually took over their hospitals' radiology departments, gaining new respect and confidence in the institutional setting.

The war effort even interrupted the professional organizations. Because of government restrictions on transportation — along with just about everything else in daily life — annual meetings of the ASXT were suspended from 1943 to 1945, but affiliate state societies were encouraged to host whatever gatherings they could as long as the meetings did not "impede or interfere with an all-out war effort by the people." To encourage increased membership, the ASXT membership committee used war bonds as an incentive, offering a bond to the affiliated society attracting the largest number of new members.

Now more than 1,900 members strong, the ASXT had reason to pause on May 6, 1943. Despite the war — or perhaps because of it and the military training programs — the American College of Radiology became a co-sponsor of the Registry with the ASXT, taking

A Good Opportunity

What of the technicians themselves and their role in the work force? In 1939 New York state conducted a thorough survey that determined 88 percent of the state's technicians were employed by hospitals. Hours worked and duties performed varied greatly. Wages ranged from a low of $50 per month with "maintenance" (basic uniforms, room and board), to $100 per month without maintenance. The head technician in a large laboratory might expect as much as $300 per month.

It is interesting to note the New York survey considered the position of x-ray technician to represent a "good opportunity."

Why? The report stated, "X-ray technicians are not greatly affected by fluctuations of the business world. The number of opportunities presented in one year is small . . . but, at the same time, there are relatively few adequately trained x-ray technicians to be found. The position of x-ray technician has many advantages and ranks higher than that of nurse or laboratory technician. It is extremely interesting to the scientifically inclined, varied and stimulating, clean, without hazard and affords the opportunity for personal achievement."

The survey was perhaps the first visible sign that "trained" x-ray technicians had begun to achieve a status worthy of acknowledgement.

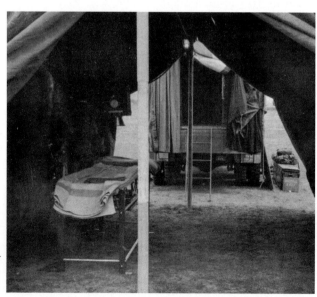

U.S. Army

Circa 1944 - *Interior view of an auxiliary mobile x-ray unit with radiographic room in foreground and darkroom in rear of truck in background.*

over the responsibilities of RSNA. This represented a new level of official recognition of the Society by physicians.

A year later, in June 1944, the AMA's Council on Medical Education and Hospitals accepted the responsibility of classifying and listing approved schools for x-ray technicians. Previously this duty had been the responsibility of the Registry. That council also took on the task of overseeing inspection of educational programs, thereby stabilizing standards so qualifications for registration might be more rigidly enforced.

The move alleviated what had been one of the ASXT's and Registry's most gnawing problems — educational standards. Despite numerous attempts in the past to establish firm educational guidelines, neither the Society nor the Registry had the wherewithal to physically police the many training courses, or the technicians graduating from them.

In 1940 there were 90 accredited programs for x-ray technicians in the United States. By 1943 more than 150 programs appeared on the Registry's approved list, with more in the application process. Yet no college education was required as a prerequisite for training. This dilemma became more serious as more radiologists showed preference for technicians with some college education.

The war did its best to bring the problem into sharper focus. While military training programs found standards endorsed by the ASXT and Registry "inadequate," there was an equal suspicion that service training was nothing more than a "mill" approach. Neither side trusted the other, and with that mistrust it was clear something had to be done.

At stake was the reputation of the Society and the Registry — both under the scrutiny of the RSNA, the AMA and the public. Despite the most severe conditions created by wartime, the Registry and the ASXT exerted their maximum effort to bring into focus

The Canadian Connection

In 1940 the x-ray technicians in the Canadian Province of Ontario decided to establish a local Registry, comparable to the ARXT. With the full cooperation of Canadian radiologists, the group invited aid from the American Registry to make their organization "comparable in procedure and effect." The long-range plan of this group called for a charter "for the entire Dominion of Canada with eventual affiliation with the British Society of Radiographers."

By 1943 the Ontario Registry was in full bloom, and the first meeting of the Canadian Society of Radiological Technicians had been held. A reciprocal agreement was reached between the Canadian and American societies for the mutual honoring of credentials and inter-society cooperation. Many Canadian technicians, however, continued to seek certification with the older and longer-established American Registry.

what needed to be done to ensure, once and for all, a future for the technicians each group served.

Higher educational standards were adopted. Gambling that the costs for potential technicians to attain higher education would not reduce the number entering the profession, the Society and Registry — both highly dependent on registration fees from applicants — waited. The gamble paid off because of the increasing demand for qualified technicians' services across a wide spectrum of medicine and industry.

By gaining AMA recognition, raising educational standards and finding that the number

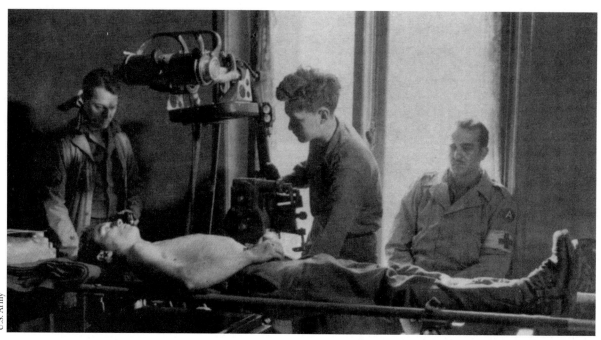

U.S. Army

Circa 1944 - *Examination of a wounded serviceman with a portable x-ray unit at the 60th Field Hospital, Nancy, France.*

of technicians seeking certification continued to increase, the Society and Registry not only persevered, they prospered. Most importantly, registered technicians achieved a higher degree of professionalism in the eyes of the medical community.

The future for technicians would have looked bright had not the war continued to expand in Europe and the Pacific.

In Europe, Col. Kenneth D. Allen, MC, served as the senior consultant in radiology for the European theater. His duties included advising personnel, procuring equipment, implementing radiation protection, supervising radiation therapy and acting as liaison with other radiology personnel in the Allied armies.

Allen insisted that radiation protection in U.S. Army hospitals in the field should be as good as civilian hospitals whenever possible. Brick partitions in combination with barium plastered walls and lead metal sheeting, when available, provided satisfactory protection for the x-ray technician. Most of the time technicians cut a small hole in the lead sheeting to peer through, instead of looking around the

corner at the patient. Lead glass was almost nonexistent in field situations.

Allen also required that films be marked regularly with the patient's name, rank, serial number, the date and hospital. The requisitioned lead letters for marking films were quickly lost, leaving technicians to make their own. Some whittled letters out of lead, others commandeered plaster of paris from the dentist and filled it with molten lead, creating a lead marker of sorts. Allen stressed the importance of keeping patients and films together, even if it meant tying the films to the patient.

Allen also recognized the need for additional radiologists and technicians throughout the field and evacuation hospitals in Europe. One hospital in Normandy had one radiologist and two technicians who worked around the clock after the invasion. Another radiologist was assigned to relieve the original doctor and to ensure the technicians were supervised at all times.

Those technicians in field hospitals usually "had less radiologic supervision and it was important that they be of the highest caliber." In field hospitals where additional radiology personnel were needed immediately, commanding officers selected the most qualified person for the job from within the group.

The United States relied heavily on the British to supply x-ray equipment and additional training of technicians and radiologists if necessary, because government restrictions prevented shipping equipment or sending troops home for training. The relationship between the U.S. and British radiology personnel was sometimes strained and competitive. Allen strove to build rapport with the British by sending American technicians and radiologists for week-long training sessions on British technique and equipment at the Royal Army Medical School. Allen was also instrumental in obtaining portable x-ray machines for the field by using the British-made MX-2.

Despite Allen's efforts, most technicians and radiologists had to improvise. In the early years of the war, chain letters circulated between hospitals. They described substitutes for cassette holders, compression bands, cones, illuminators and dryers, and were accompanied by photos, designs and sometimes an actual model.

In the Pacific theater, radiologists and x-ray technicians received little if any guidance from senior consultants in Oahu, Hawaii. X-ray technicians were in short supply throughout the region. Most were transferred from hospitals to combat units.

Requests for replacements often were answered with "Train your own." The Trippler Hospital on Oahu started a program lasting from six weeks to seven months depending on the combat situation. The technicians also were trained in clerical and darkroom duties. All medical personnel and supplies were in such demand that during extreme conditions, the Army and Navy would exchange patients, personnel and supplies to cover the shortage.

Equipment — if technicians could get their hands on it — was usually substandard and outdated. One unit had open overhead cables and Coolidge tubes with lead enclosures. Other medical units were sometimes fortunate to get Portable X-ray Unit Number 91085, otherwise known as the "Workhorse."

Improvisation became the norm. "X-ray technicians were ingenious men, and their ingenuity, based on observation and experience, helped to overcome shortages and lack of adequate equipment. They often seemed, in fact, to take delight in surmounting obstacles unknown in civilian life." Shell casings made great cones and troubleshooting equipment problems became a valuable skill.

The hospitals along the northern coast of New Guinea were well-equipped with radiographic equipment, even down to a tilting table in one Navy hospital. The larger facilities were equipped with 10 to 15 milliampere

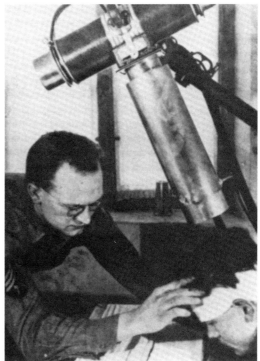

Circa 1944 - *An Army radiographer from the 36th General Hospital in Caserta, Italy, improvises an extension cylinder using a shell casing attached to a Picker field unit.*

portable equipment, but the activity was restricted to a few basic procedures. The reason: as many as 300 wounded might arrive on any given day.

Aside from a shortage of x-ray film because of the isolated locations, weather and distance in the tropics made x-ray work difficult. A major technical hazard was fluctuating electrical power. In the time it took to change plates, a power fluctuation of 50 percent variation in exposure was common. High temperatures and humidity also made film handling difficult. Open film had to be stored in dry containers, and special developing and fixing techniques were used. Hospitals were constantly being moved. Trying to install refrigerating tanks was useless.

Back on the home front, shortages of just about everything became critical, and great emphasis was placed on what could be salvaged or reused. Discarded radiographs and spoiled x-ray film were stripped of emulsion and attached to windowpanes to increase the strength of the glass in the event of a bomb-induced concussion.

The Military Committee of the RSNA published a letter calling on radiologists to "use sparingly and with great care the x-ray equipment and accessories on hand, such as cassettes, intensifying screens, developing hangers and tanks, x-ray tubes, x-ray meters and film driers."

In late 1944 x-ray film was rationed again. Technicians sometimes used x-ray paper instead of film for gastrointestinal and colon examinations. This was done, according to the July 1945 issue of *The X-Ray Technician*, on thin patients mostly "though we did make one six-hour gastrointestinal checkup on a 295-pound patient just to prove that it could be done." Though considerable adaptation of exposure times was required and the paper tended to curl, technicians achieved satisfactory results.

Technology Marches On

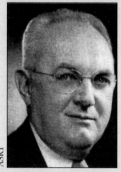

Arthur W. Fuchs

Arthur Fuchs, son of Wolfram Conrad Fuchs, electrician from the Cicero and Proviso Railroad who later founded the Fuchs X-Ray Laboratory, developed the optimum voltage technique — involving the wavelength of Roentgen rays necessary to penetrate tissue.

During World War II, while serving as chief of the X-Ray Section, School for Medical Department, Technicians, Army Medical Center, Fuchs refined the technique by using it on military personnel. But because of the essential uniformity of patients — between 18 and 40 years old — the technique did not adapt well to the civilian world. Regardless, Fuchs was responsible for training hundreds of technicians during the war.

Other developments during the war included introduction of the Filmachine, a mechanical film processor designed to serve high volume x-ray laboratories. During the war the Filmachine was also used by the military for processing x-rays inspecting military related products.

The betatron was also developed during the war. Utilizing electrons, the machine had a 3.5 ton magnet and weighed more than 4 tons complete, although the unit was no larger than a regular office desk. Designed to generate a powerful x-ray beam, the betatron was capable of producing a stream of electrons at 20 million volts.

Everything was in short supply. The ASXT was asked by the government to reduce the number of pages of its journal to help the nation conserve paper. Technicians were even requested to save the interleafing paper from x-ray films for donation to the national drive for scrap paper.

But as difficult as the war years were, forward-thinking members of the Registry and ASXT posed another question: What would happen when the war ended and military x-ray technicians returned to civilian life?

The Registry expressed its concern over how to "sift" the service-trained technicians, and suggested that all technicians keep accurate records of their work and supervision, securing the necessary documentation from their medical officers. At a September 1944 meeting of the ASXT Council on Education and Registration, members recommended careful evaluation of the training received by Armed Forces technicians before they be considered for registration.

By the end of the war, 9,000 men had been trained by the military as x-ray technicians. The Registry boasted a total of 5,500 registered technicians. It was estimated that 20,000 x-ray installations were functioning in civilian medical practice, many of which were operated by owner-physicians, some of whom were not radiologists.

The ASXT posed the following dilemma: "Looking to the future, the immediate postwar period will see thousands of x-ray technicians released from military service and wartime jobs. Of these thousands, many will probably make an effort to take a place in this profession as civilians. Quite possibly, many of these... will not bring to the profession the technical skill or the ethical bearing that will be advantageous to their associates.

"Their presence will bring the type of publicity which will tend to lower the profession in the estimate of the medical world and give a false impression to the layman. Even now it would be well to take the ethical and legitimate steps necessary to establish the x-ray technical profession and the registered technician on a high plane, so that if and when unfavorable incidents are attributed to members of this profession, (the public) may know the differentiating circumstances between the registered... and the non-registered technician."

Was this just more paranoia? Yes and no. As hard as the ASXT and Registry had fought for professional recognition, even a small incident carried repercussions. A case in point: A 1943 article in the *Chicago Daily News* (later reprinted in the Society's journal) told of an incident concerning a "devil-dancer" — a young woman "who spent her days as a student x-ray technician in one Chicago hospital while her nights were occu-

Better Safe Than Sorry

In 1943 the Advisory Committee on X-Ray and Radium Protection published a pamphlet containing a unified set of safety recommendations, including the proper use of filters, the location of x-ray rooms and their appropriate protective lining of lead or other suitable material.

To test for scatter radiation, it was suggested workers clip a dental film on their pockets for two weeks. If the developed film showed the image of the clip, then more protection was needed. Later, it was suggested that a film wrapped in black paper to prevent fogging from ordinary light be fixed in position where the test was to be made, and if after 10 days the film was less than black the worker needed to take additional precautions. This was the first radiation protection badge.

The Issue of Race

In the 1930s it was rare for African Americans to be trained at approved schools. Not until St. Mary's Infirmary in St. Louis, Mo., began to accept minority patients did things change. William E. Allen Jr. was appointed radiologist in chief and he, with Sisters Mary Alacoque Anger, R.T., and Mary Fides Stolz, R.T., organized a school for African American students. However, students were restricted to young, unmarried females — the same restrictions found at the school of nursing.

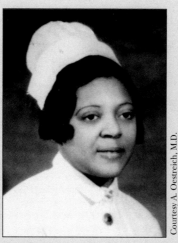

Rose Marie Pegues

Courtesy A. Oestreich, M.D.

The first African American registered as an x-ray technician was Rose M. Pegues, R.T., R.N., who was trained at St. Mary's School. Although there was initial resistance to Pegues taking the exam, a united effort (led by Sister Mary Alacoque) overcame the bias, and Pegues passed the exam in 1936.

In the East, one of the early schools for minority x-ray technicians was established by James L. Morton in 1937 at Freedman's Hospital in Washington, D.C. This school grew through the years and became accredited in 1963. In 1946 William Allen Jr. established another x-ray technology school at St. Louis' Homer G. Phillips Hospital.

Allen's school had no restrictions regarding age, sex or marital status. Class size averaged 10 students, with 20 in training. After graduation of the first class on Sept. 10, 1948, the school rapidly gained in enrollment. By the 1960s it graduated approximately 200 black radiographers, nuclear medicine technologists and radiation therapists.

Allen would also be the first African American radiologist to volunteer for active military service. Allen was eventually assigned to a station hospital in Fort Huachuca, Ariz., staffed by minority medical officers. This facility later grew into a 1,500-bed Ninth Service Command Regional Hospital, where Allen trained medical officers in elementary roentgenology.

Allen also established the first and only African American women's Army Corps School for X-Ray Technologists. The majority of the hospital's permanent staff qualified for the exams of the ARRT and became registered.

But becoming registered was only the beginning battle for African Americans. These technicians were denied membership in many technologist societies, so they formed their own, the earliest in 1940 being the Mound City Society of X-Ray Technologists in St. Louis.

– Paul Young

pied in tripping the light fantastic in special routines at a night club.

"According to the writer, the dancing 'roentgenologist' was to graduate within a few weeks 'from a training course at the hospital with the title Registered Technician.' The whole incident might have passed as just another humorous 'working girl' story had not the writer chosen to use the terms 'roentgenologist and registered technician.' Needless to say, the 'devil-dancer' was summarily dismissed from the training program by the radiologist-in-charge, who 'courteously

expressed regrets for the implications cast by this unfortunate incident.'"

A small, seemingly insignificant event, yet one that pointed out "technicians are made to realize that they are not always in control of the circumstances leading up to situations which may prove to be disastrous to the x-ray technical profession."

Simpler times, under difficult circumstances.

Had the ASXT and the Registry prepared themselves for what was coming?

Portrait of an R.T.

Theodore Ott completed his R.T. training in the Navy and, after establishing a radiological department at the Norfolk Navy Yard in Portsmouth, found himself on board the rescue ship, USS PCER (Patrol Craft Emergency Rescue), in the Pacific theater. The duty of the ship was to transport injured soldiers to a waiting hospital ship.

Ott says he worked with x-ray equipment that fit in three suitcases, alongside an orthopedic surgeon fresh from medical school. "Neither of us had ever seen so many wounded Marines. We would go onto the beaches, many times under enemy gunfire, to determine who was salvageable. We did triage on the beach."

After the Japanese surrendered, Ott's ship was one of four commissioned to deactivate some 90,000 pressure sensitive mines hidden in the Japan inland sea. The lead boat was a patched freighter used to bring the mines to the surface. Boats 2 and 3 were "sweepers" — one port side, one starboard of the freighter — that deactivated the mines by detonating or sinking them.

Ott's boat followed behind as an emergency medical facility in case of casualties, of which there was only one. A soldier was struck on the back of the head by falling shrapnel from an exploding mine.

Not all of Ott's memories of the war were bad, though. He recalled one instance while in the northern Pacific when "one of the seamen fell overboard into the cold water. He was pulled out shivering and the doctor said, 'Get this man down under and give him a shot of bourbon!' Back then, bourbon and medicinal alcohol were rationed and sometimes used for barter to get medical supplies from the Army. Within the next hour, four other men had 'fallen' overboard — any-

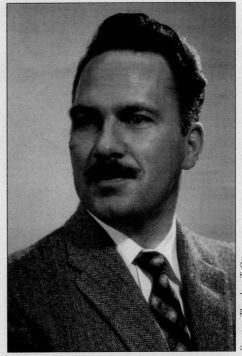

Theodore Ott served as an x-ray technician in the Pacific during World War II.

thing for a shot of bourbon!"

During the tour in the Japan sea, Ott visited Hiroshima three weeks after the atomic bomb was dropped.

"There were only four building structures standing — a Baptist church, the city hall, the newspaper building and one other. Even bricks were blown to bits. I saw a trolley car that looked like it had been clapped between two giant hands," he recalled.

After the war, Ott worked at the Los Angeles County General Hospital as senior technician, and eventually joined the staff of the UCLA Medical Center as technical director of the radiology department. Later he was named radiology administrator there.

Active in both the California and the national societies, Ott has been an ASRT fellow since 1964.

– Barbara Pongracz-Bartha

Chapter Seven

The Emergence of Excellence

World War II concluded in as dramatic a fashion as it had begun. Using the atomic bomb to force Japan's surrender not only ended the war, but also heralded the beginning of a new era in which technology emerged as the single most powerful force in the world's future. In the medical profession, the atomic age ushered in an expanding interest in the use of radioisotopes to both diagnose and treat disease. And just as the development of sonar during World War II inspired the science of sonography, the unleashing of nuclear power spawned new medical techniques.

This age of technological specialization would create a prosperity even the optimism of America could not have foreseen. The ASXT and the Registry, which persevered through the Great Depression and World War II, now could reap the benefits of their determination and turn their attention to promoting new standards of excellence for the profession.

Despite Alfred Greene's fears of 9,000 returning military-trained technicians overwhelming the civilian work force, a great majority chose other pursuits. A few entered industry, where the x-ray was finding wider use in quality control and product develop-

ment. Veterans whose interests remained in medicine obtained further education and pursued their Registry certificates. Because of the continuing shortage in the number of registered technicians, they were not dissuaded. In fact, a March 1947 article in *The X-Ray Technician* titled "From G.I. to R.T." encouraged veterans to consider careers in radiography. "Men, and especially women, coming back from military duty and wondering where to start a new life should be informed by their rehabilitation officers about the profession of x-ray technician," the writer advised. "In my opinion, the work of an x-ray technician is fascinating enough to attract and hold the most unsettled veteran who has any ambition for professional achievement and satisfaction."

Under the G.I. Bill, the student veteran could receive a monthly stipend of $65 if single or $95 if married. Because the profession was dominated by women, female students were preferred, giving women who served in the Army and Navy an advantage at becoming x-ray technicians. By 1946 the AMA's Council on Medical Education and Hospitals had approved 130 schools for x-ray technicians, with a capacity of about 620 students. Average tuition for one year ran about $45.

In 1945 the Registry reported the number

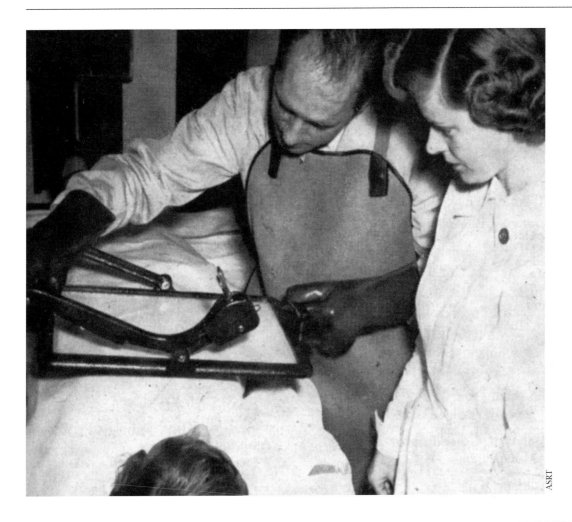

ASRT

1952 - (top) Despite an intense effort by the ASXT, many x-ray technicians still did not practice radiation safety. In this photo, the radiologist is protected, but the technician is not.

Circa 1951 - (right) Devices designed to improve exposure technique, as represented by this advertisement for a hand held "technic computer," helped standardize x-ray procedures in the 1940s and '50s.

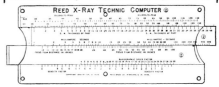

of new applicants at 453, an 18 percent increase over the previous year. As anticipated, the majority were veterans. In fact, the ARXT registered more technicians during the five-year period from 1945 to 1950 than it had during its previous 23 years of existence. By 1950, registered technicians totaled more than 7,500.

Much of the credit for the Registry's growth during this period goes to Alfred Greene. Incredible as it may seem, Greene operated the burgeoning Registry for many years while continuing to work full-time as an x-ray technician. As early as 1934 Greene wore four different hats, serving simultaneously as executive secretary of the Registry, secretary-treasurer of the ASXT, editor of *The X-Ray Technician* and chief x-ray technician at the Glen Lake Sanatorium outside Minneapolis. Initially, Greene operated the Registry out of a dug-out crawl space beneath one of the sanatorium's buildings.

By 1941 the increased level of Registry business forced Greene to resign his position at Glen Lake and move the Registry office into a spare bedroom in his apartment. With this change, Greene became the Registry's first full-time employee.

With the surge in the number of registered technicians following World War II, the Registry Board agreed to purchase a house in Minneapolis for Greene with the understanding that the Registry offices would occupy space on its second floor. However, even that space soon was outgrown and Registry operations overflowed into the entire house, including the basement and garage. So, in 1950, the Registry underwrote the addition of a dormer on the house. Greene's wife, Rose, must have been incredibly patient and tolerant.

By 1955 the Registry board approved the rental of space in an office building in downtown Minneapolis to house the growing Registry office, which for the first time would not have to share space with another organization or the Greene household.

As each successive year brought increasing numbers of technicians wishing to be registered, the ARXT gradually realized its examination process had to become more efficient. For the first 25 years of the Registry's existence, applicants had to complete a two-part examination — a theoretical exam consisting of essay-type questions and a practical exam that required the submission of a series of x-rays demonstrating specific techniques. In January 1952 the Registry board reduced the number of essay-type questions and added objective, multiple-choice questions to the exam for the first time. In November 1954 the board stopped requiring the submission of sample x-rays as part of the exam. And in May 1955 the Registry moved to an entirely multiple-choice format for its exam to keep up with the growing number of examinees. This new exam format could be scored by machine, thus making results available earlier.

This period of unprecedented growth for the Registry was not without its occasional challenges. In fact, the Registry was forced to re-evaluate many of its regulations during the 1940s and '50s. For example, when the Registry was originally formed, anyone who had two years of on-the-job experience in the technical aspects of x-ray work and could obtain a physician's recommendation was considered eligible to take the national registration exam. Unfortunately, these broad eligibility requirements reinforced some physicians' perceptions of x-ray technicians as mere "button-pushers" with no special education or training. A 1942 article in *The X-Ray Technician* stated the problem succinctly:

"Sad to say, too often x-ray technicians and button-pushers are confused in the minds of many. It is granted that equipment manufacturers have come a long way toward the elim-

90 Seconds After the Ball of Fire

The birth of the atomic age in 1945 signaled the end of World War II, but the modern spectre of nuclear warfare brought new threats of world domination and spawned the Cold War between the United States and the Soviet Union. The proliferation of nuclear weapons in the 1950s and the threat of Communism fostered paranoia in every facet of American society. Fears of the atomic bomb — and, later, the hydrogen bomb and the intercontinental ballistic missile — led President Dwight D. Eisenhower to label the decade between 1950 and 1960 "the age of peril."

Radiographers' concerns about the Cold War and the threat of nuclear attack were evident as articles titled "Medical Aspects of an Atomic Explosion," "The X-Ray Technician and the Atomic Bomb" and "Civil Defense and You" began appearing in the ASXT journal in the early 1950s.

In 1950 ASXT President John Cahoon, R.T., offered the Society's services to the Atomic Bomb Casualty Commission and the War Department "in the event of a national emergency." A year later, the ASXT created its own Committee on Civil Defense. The committee's reports during the next several years included thoughts on what would happen if a hospital were hit, how many technicians would be lost, and how many technicians in outlying areas should be trained in emergency procedures.

Because they were familiar with the properties of x-radiation, technicians were encouraged to learn how to recognize radiation sickness to deal with problems likely to arise from a nuclear detonation. In fact, many believed that x-ray technicians and radiologists would take on vital roles during an atomic war. An article by James Wick, R.T., in the March 1950 issue of *The X-Ray*

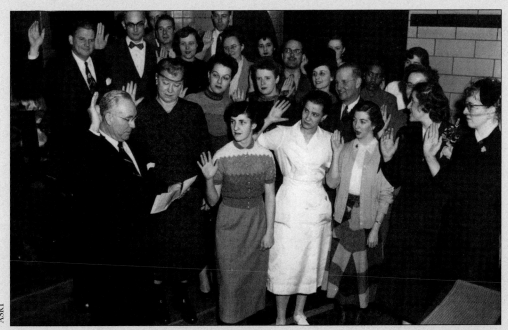

ASRT

Circa 1953 - *Members of the Philadelphia Society of X-Ray Technicians were sworn into the Civilian Defense Program.*

Technician warned that the next world war would be a "radiological war" and that x-ray technicians should prepare themselves. "In the event of such a war, our government has plans for a radiological defense of every city," Wick wrote. "Who would head such a defense in your city? Certainly, the radiologist. Whom would he ask to be his assistants in training of the population for defense against this type of warfare? Without question, it would be his technicians."

In a 1951 editorial, committee member Richard Olden, R.T., encouraged fellow x-ray technicians to learn all they could about atomic warfare and prepare themselves for its aftermath. "Each of you has probably asked yourself how you, as an x-ray technician, can best serve in the event of a major catastrophe or atomic bombing," he wrote. "As technicians, we have a considerable responsibility. The majority of casualties resulting from an atomic attack will undoubtedly require first aid or hospitalization. Technicians will be required to examine many of these patients radiographically... (and) use radiation detection equipment (or) instruct others in the use of this equipment." Olden added, "This is not a problem to be treated with complacency. We must be prepared and we must prepare now — tomorrow may be too late. Civil defense is everybody's business!" He urged every ASXT member to volunteer for community civil defense training.

On May 7-8, 1951, members of the ASXT Committee on Civil Defense joined representatives of 300 other organizations in Washington, D.C., for a special conference on emergency preparedness. President Harry S Truman addressed the attendees, reminding them that national defense efforts would require the "combined, unselfish work" of "many hundreds of thou-

sands of private citizens."

As the Civil Defense phenomenon reached near-hysteria proportions, misinformation often was the rule of thumb. Newspaper reporters falsely reassured the public by publishing erroneous data based on inconclusive research. The ASXT's own journal, *The X-Ray Technician*, was no exception. One article appearing in January 1952 advised readers that "heavy clothing will give fair protection" from radioactive fallout and "36 inches of concrete will protect a person from radiation when under the explosion; 20 inches of concrete will give protection if one is a half-mile from the explosion and only two inches at one mile."

In a lecture at the 1950 Iowa Society of X-Ray Technicians annual meeting, one technician urged his colleagues not to let concerns about the radiation effects of an atomic bomb prevent them from administering first aid. "When the atomic bomb goes off, many of the fissionable products are radioactive. The resulting rays are dangerous, as you have learned in the popular press. But what the press has not emphasized is that the decay period is only the time it takes to blink your eyes twice.

"This means that by the time you have recovered from the shock of the attack, the fire blast and shock wave, the danger of irradiation will already have done its damage and it will be safe for you to get away from the area, or go into the area to assist in rescue work. The latest time recommendation is 90 seconds after the ball of fire. Remember! Should an atomic attack come into the area in which you happen to be and you are not in your predetermined disaster position or post, do not let the bugaboo of irradiation fear prevent you from saving yourself and some other human."

—*Ceela McElveny*

ination of many knobs and buttons on the control panel, and x-ray equipment these days carries more automatic and fool-proof devices than in an earlier period, but so long as the individual patient remains the causative factor behind an x-ray examination, x-ray pictures will not be easy to make…. It is precisely to dissipate this prevalent fallacy that x-ray technicians are making definite steps towards limiting this field to those better qualified by training and educational background."

These steps included stiffening eligibility requirements for certification by the Registry. The new requirements, which went into effect in July 1942, stated that to become certified a technician had to prove that he or she had a high school diploma or its equivalent and had two years of experience under the direction of a radiologist or four years of experience under the supervision of any other type of physician. In 1951 this requirement was changed again, with Registry applicants having to prove one year of experience served directly under the supervision of a radiologist.

Another long-standing requirement was that applicants had to be at least 21 years old to take the Registry exam. In the years after the war, however, students and some educators began questioning this age restriction. They argued that prospective technicians who finished high school at age 17 and completed their education in x-ray technology by 19 were not eligible to take the Registry exam for two more years.

The minimum age requirement was a divisive topic at Registry board meetings in the late 1940s. During a 1947 meeting, Registry Trustee John Keichline, M.D., noted that "Down in Georgia the law is that boys and girls at the age of 18 can vote. If in Georgia they are allowed to vote at 18, why of course I don't see why we could not take them into the Registry at 19."

But others disagreed. Erminda Clarke, R.T., the first female member of the Registry board and a former ASXT president, responded, "We feel that the age of 21 years and the judgment that goes with it are necessary before the technician makes up his mind that x-ray technique is the field he wants to enter… If the Society and the College want to lower it to 19, then lower the standards and abide by them… but don't blame the Registry board because you have registered technicians too young to do the work that you feel registration should give them the knowledge to do."

Despite Clarke's warning, the Registry — under continued pressure from younger students — in November 1949 amended its bylaws to drop the minimum age limit and accept applicants younger than 21, provided they met the other eligibility requirements.

Another challenge for the Registry arose when technicians began asking for special credentials as a way to recognize additional education or experience. The idea of a designation of "master technician" to distinguish superior qualifications first appeared in the mid-1930s, but it resurfaced with a vengeance in the 1950s. "Why can't the ARXT set up a post-graduate program for R.T.s in which additional education and ability will be recognized and honored by additional exams?" one technician asked during an open forum with the Registry board at the 1950 ASXT Annual Conference.

At the time, both the Registry and the Society were opposed to additional certification, arguing that registration alone was sufficient. "We can all be proud that we are R.T.s and not ask for anything else," one Registry board member said, temporarily putting the issue to rest. "The R.T. needs no further recognition."

External forces also had an impact on the Registry. In 1956 a new registry group for technicians attempted to organize in Enid, Okla. Calling itself the American Radiogra-

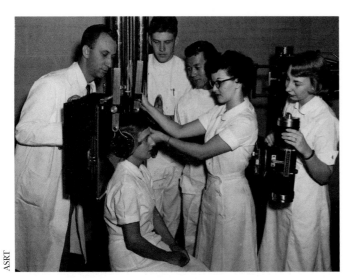

The class of 1952 from Johns Hopkins Hospital's x-ray technology program demonstrate their skills for Richard Olden (left), their program director.

phy Technologists, this group tried to draw x-ray technicians away from the ARXT, threatening to splinter the profession. The ARXT fought back against what it called the "pseudo-Registry," filing papers in Washington, D.C., for exclusive rights to the term "registered technician." In the end, the competing group failed because it could not withstand the withering condemnation of the American College of Radiology, which stood firmly by its support of the ARXT.

However, the threat represented by the splinter organization could not be ignored. As the use of radioisotopes in medicine expanded in the 1950s, the Registry realized that it had to reach out to nuclear medicine and radiation therapy technicians or risk losing them to organizations outside radiology. As a result, the ARXT began considering separate exams for radiation therapy technicians and "isotope technicians" in 1955, although these exams were not instituted until nearly a decade later.

By 1956 close to 15,000 technicians were registered with the ARXT. Its numbers had almost doubled in just six years.

Naturally, the increasing number of registered technicians was paralleled by increased membership in the ASXT. Throughout the 1940s, the number of registered technicians who also were members of the ASXT hovered between 40 and 50 percent. In 1948 the ASXT boasted 2,589 members (44.5 percent of registered technicians); in 1952 ASXT membership reached 4,207 (42.3 percent of those registered). The Society's leaders, of course, believed that 100 percent of registered technicians should be members of the professional organization, and accordingly launched a massive membership campaign in the late 1940s. Its theme was "Every R.T. a member of ASXT," and the campaign succeeded in increasing Society membership by nearly 20 percent between the years of 1948 and 1949.

Despite the growth in the number of technicians, many hospital x-ray departments found themselves short-handed. Demand for trained x-ray technicians, which first peaked in the early 1940s, continued unabated into the early '50s. Richard Olden, R.T., president of the Society from 1953-54, made meeting

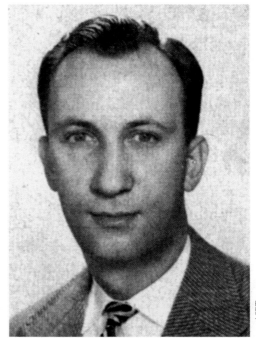

1952 - Richard Olden, R.T., ASXT president.

"the existing demands for qualified x-ray technologists" one of his top priorities. "This cannot be accomplished unless additional students are induced to enter the field of x-ray technology," he noted. As a result, the Society developed a recruitment brochure for the profession and distributed it to high schools throughout the country.

One innovative solution to the personnel shortage was "The Philadelphia Plan" — a 25-month x-ray training program conducted jointly by local high schools and four area hospitals. When the first class of 16 students graduated on March 20, 1953, every graduate found immediate work in the profession. At the following year's graduation ceremony, one radiologist remarked on the necessity of programs such as the Philadelphia Plan to ease the severe technician shortage.

"There are at present more than 300 approved schools of x-ray technology in 43 states, but the turnout of graduate technicians is still too small to meet pressing needs for their services," he said. "Unless the number of students entering training increases substantially — and soon — we will face such a shortage of x-ray technicians that it will hamstring institutions, hospitals, health services, industry and teaching programs, not to speak of radiologists in private practice."

With pressure mounting to recruit increasing numbers of technicians, the need for educational standards for the profession became obvious. As early as 1937, a survey by Sister Mary Alacoque Anger, R.T., found a lack of uniformity concerning the quality of educational programs and their curricula. Ten years later, the situation had changed little. In fact, an informal survey of accredited x-ray technician schools in 1946 showed that the majority kept no records of students' clinical experiences.

There also was great variation in the length of educational programs offered by these institutions. Of the schools of x-ray technology approved by the AMA's Council on Medical Education and Hospitals in 1947, 103 offered a one-year training program — the minimum acceptable — while 19 had a course lasting 18 months and 34 had two-year programs. All courses were presented in hospitals, although 51 were affiliated with colleges or universities.

With technology expanding and technical requirements changing rapidly, ASXT leaders knew that this array of educational programs somehow had to be standardized. The Society began seriously investigating a basic minimum curriculum for the profession in the early 1950s, turning the issue over to its Education Committee. By 1952 the committee had developed a model standardized curriculum and submitted it to the American College of Radiology for approval.

Explaining the committee's thoughts in designing the curriculum, member Richard Olden noted, "There is little uniformity in the program of our training schools throughout the country.... In evaluating the essentials for standardization, it was realized that the first step was to select the subjects essential in preparing students for radiographic work. It was then necessary to weigh the importance of each of these subjects, list them in logical sequence and estimate the number of hours to be devoted to each one. In this manner, we have attempted to establish certain requirements for a basic minimum curriculum."

The curriculum proposed by the Society was approved by the ACR in October 1952. It described a one-year course in x-ray technology, although the Society noted that a two-year educational program was preferred. The curriculum recommended 30 hours of positioning and clinical practice, 20 hours of physics, 20 hours of anatomy and physiology, 10 hours of darkroom technique, 10 hours of x-ray technique, 10 hours of special procedures, 10 hours of nursing procedures, five hours of radiation safety, five hours of office procedures, five hours of radiation therapy, three hours of department administration, two hours of ethics, two hours of medical terminology and weekly film critique sessions. Although the ASXT strongly recommended its adoption by educational programs, no requirement that this curriculum be followed was included in the *Essentials* of an approved school. Actually improving education standards for the technician, therefore, continued to be a thorny problem.

In addition to boosting the quality of educational programs at x-ray schools, the Society continued to emphasize education at its own Annual Conference. Its efforts won the admiration of K.D. Allen, M.D., president of the Registry Board of Trustees. After attending the 1948 ASXT Annual Conference, Allen wrote, "Seldom has anyone seen a more earnest group regularly attending early morning sessions with the obvious desire to improve their knowledge of radiography, x-ray physics and necessary anatomy. Any group which conducts such a meeting, with practically no time given to any subjects other than scientific ones, cannot be called anything but a professional group."

In 1955 the Society introduced the "Workshop Day," a full day of educational programming that became increasingly popular at annual meetings. The Society also published a guide to educational aids, titled "Training Aids for Schools of X-Ray Technology," that listed 250 motion pictures, 25 film strips and more than 80 recommended textbooks.

Despite the Society's emphasis on technician education, the profession still had to contend with inconsistent hospital hiring policies. Hospitals did not always give special consideration to registered technicians, who naturally expected better financial compensation based on their educational achievements. And even though the AMA was committed to program accreditation, physicians themselves sometimes did not advocate hiring the most qualified candidate because even into the 1950s it was common for the salary of the hospital technician to be paid by a radiologist with privileges at the hospital. The Society, nevertheless, continued to push for uniform educational standards for technicians, believing they eventually would lead to increased status for the profession.

The Society's efforts to standardize technician education also were an effective counterstrategy to the state licensure movement of the era. The ASXT had long remained staunch in its opposition to three issues: unionization, socialized medicine and state licensure. Of the three, the Society believed licensure represented the biggest threat to the profession as a whole.

The licensure issue first arose in 1937 in Kentucky, where state legislators passed a bill to license x-ray technicians. The bill later was ruled unconstitutional by the attorney general and declared null and void. During the next decade, similar licensure bills were attempted in South Carolina, Pennsylvania, New York, Oklahoma, Washington, California and Connecticut, all without success.

The ASXT opposed state licensure because it believed nationwide registration through the ARXT was more effective. During a panel discussion at the 1948 Annual Conference in Minneapolis, speakers argued licensure would "legislate technicians out of their jobs" and "reduce all technicians in the state to a common level of mediocrity by offering the finest technicians in the state a credential no better than that available to the most incompetent part-time button-pusher."

Furthermore, the ACR opposed state licensure and strongly advised the ASXT to work against it. ACR Executive Director Mac Cahal,

A Home in Fond du Lac

Some people seem to have been born for special roles in life. Genevieve Eilert, R.T., was one of them. The unusual coincidence between her professional interests and her hometown brought the ASXT into the little Wisconsin burg of Fond du Lac in the late 1930s, where it remained for more than 20 years and matured under Eilert's guidance.

Genevieve Eilert practically was raised as a child of radiologic technology. She learned about the profession from a physician treating her for a childhood cold, and while still a teenager began training with Fond du Lac radiologist J. Rhodes Longley, M.D. After six months of x-ray studies and graduation from high school in June 1925, she went to work for Longley and, later, his associate Robert L. Waffle, M.D.

Eilert passed her Registry exam in 1931 and joined the ASXT in 1935, with a desire to contribute matched by few others. By 1937 Eilert landed the prestigious assignment as program chairman for the ASXT national convention and was elected vice president of the Society's Board of Directors. The following year she was named secretary-treasurer.

In those days the ASXT Board was elected by Society members who attended the Annual Conference. The leadership included a president, first and second vice president, secretary-treasurer and three other directors. There was no paid staff or established business office, and the Board accomplished the Society's duties simply by rolling up its collective sleeves.

Of course, it was not quite that simple. The secretary-treasurer bore the brunt of

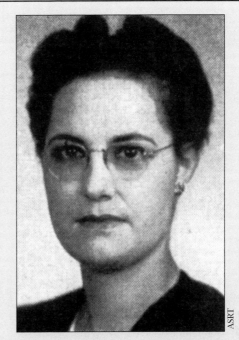

Genevieve J. Eilert

the details, essentially functioning as the Society's workhorse. General business matters were sent to the secretary-treasurer's home address, which tended to ensure longevity of service in that position.

Eilert kept all the ASXT membership applications and records, information requests, annual meeting files and general correspondence in a makeshift office in the den of her home. The Society reimbursed her for nominal expenses such as postage, supplies and telephone calls.

In the mid-1940s the ASXT formed an Executive Committee that provided improved operational stability. Eilert was named executive secretary in 1946 and became the Society's first full-time employee. She continued for the next 16 years to maintain the Society's records from her den, which also often served as meeting space for the ASXT Board.

But it couldn't last. As the 1950s came to an end, the ASXT found its membership topping 8,600 and the Society's records filled the corners and covered the floor in the Eilert family's once-cozy den. The Registry listed almost 30,000 technicians on its rolls. The profession was in full stride. Something had to be done.

In September 1962 ASXT headquarters were relocated into actual business offices at 537 Main Street in Fond du Lac. The offices were modest — although Eilert considered them "pretentious." They were located at street level around the corner from a drugstore, with three rooms serving 11 workers during the next six years.

Eilert remained in charge, overseeing a staff that handled book orders, finances, membership, state affiliate events and the activities of the national Society. Like Alfred Greene, her counterpart at the Registry, Eilert never seemed overwhelmed with her many tasks; she also served as associate editor of *The X-Ray Technician* during this time.

Her hard work paid off — though in a way she may not have expected. By 1968 ASRT members numbered 14,000, and the leadership felt the need for another step forward for the association. With the majority of radiology organizations already established in nearby Chicago, it seemed natural that the Society move there too.

Eilert and her staff, whose ties were too strong to Fond du Lac, chose not to relocate to Chicago. Eilert did help with the transition, however, commuting to Chicago during the week and returning to Fond du Lac on weekends for the first three months.

It was a difficult change for one who had been such a devoted caretaker through the years. After the Society settled in Chicago and hired its first non-technician executive, Eilert said she lost contact with many of her old organization friends. Of course, she maintained her membership and conduct-

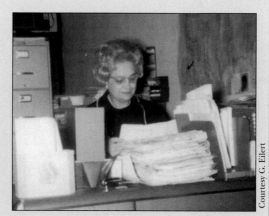

Courtesy G. Eilert

Genevieve Eilert in the Fond du Lac office.

ed occasional interviews about ASRT's early history.

Looking back on her service to the Society, Eilert said it was like being part of a big, close family. "It was just the way it was. I was dedicated and organized to a fault," she said. Her husband started working for ASXT in 1950, handling the educational materials including textbook orders and educational finances. "I was glad to do it. My husband and I worked together. It was very definitely worth it despite the sacrifices, because ASRT grew."

Annual membership dues were $3 when Eilert started as secretary-treasurer. They rose to $5 and then $10 while she was executive secretary.

Eilert said the move to Chicago altered the sense of family that she enjoyed about the Society. Recalling one incident in particular, she said, "I came into the office one day shortly after the move to find a secretary throwing away a 12-inch book of membership applications from the early days of the Society. They didn't realize what would be valuable in years to come and what was important to technologists at that time."

—Barbara Pongracz-Bartha

J.D., delivered the following warning to ASXT leaders in 1946: "If your national society or any of its affiliated state bodies actually sponsor (state licensure proposals), I believe I can assure you that the cooperative and cordial relationship that presently exists between your group and ours would be destroyed." Cahal added, "I personally think it would be a mistake to weaken the influence of the American Registry of X-Ray Technicians by substituting a governmental board for your own national board."

As a result, a resolution was passed at the Society's 1948 Annual Conference denouncing state licensure as "detrimental to the welfare of persons engaged in the profession of x-ray technology" and reaffirming the ASXT's support of the Registry as "the most economical, fair and unbiased method of establishing the qualifications of x-ray technicians."

One of the pro-licensure movement's strongest arguments was that licensure would provide a way for states to control unaccredited x-ray schools. To invalidate this argument, the ASXT proposed a more acceptable and unified standard of operation for schools offering x-ray programs, calling for period inspection of these schools by radiologists. In 1951 the ACR accepted this duty and the licensure issue stepped back into the shadows — at least temporarily.

Despite uncertainty over licensure and educational levels, many other benefits came the profession's way between 1945 and 1960, bringing security, safety and standardization to the x-ray technician's job. In February 1947 the U.S. Congress finally enacted House Resolution 1992, extending Social Security benefits to technicians employed in religious, charitable, scientific and educational institutions. Passage of this legislation was a great achievement for the ASXT, whose members had lobbied long and hard to earn this basic benefit.

Methods of measuring the amount of radia-tion to which x-ray workers were exposed also took a major step forward during this era. The majority of technicians were well aware of the damage done to their predecessors. So lead shielding and tight coning were the orders of the day, although professional commitment still caused many to forego their own safety interests for the benefit of their patients.

By the mid-1950s, the old method of clipping a dental film to a technician's pocket was replaced with commercially-produced radiation monitoring badges. These badges were processed by their manufacturer after being worn a requisite number of days. The badge company kept a permanent record for each technician and provided the employer with regular reports on radiation exposure levels. The National Committee for Radiation Protection created the concept of "permissible" whole body exposure in 1948, establishing it at 15 rem per year for occupational exposure. In 1958 the limit was lowered to 12 rem per year and in 1962 it was decreased to 5 rem per year.

Another major improvement was the establishment of standardized processing methods. Previously, technicians had to hand-process x-ray films by immersing them in individual tanks of developer and fixer solution, rinsing them in water and hanging them up to dry. Some x-ray technicians even were responsible for mixing processing chemistry. This time-consuming method often resulted in inconsistent film quality, which in turn resulted in high repeat rates.

The hand-processing tradition ended in the early 1940s with the introduction of the automatic film processor. The first of these machines used conveyor belts to move x-ray films through the developer, fixer and dryer. The cycle time for one film was about 40 minutes with the earliest models of these machines, but by the mid-1950s, manufacturers had developed roller-transport processors that could deliver a dry radiograph in only 6 minutes. The advent of automatic film processing brought tremendous changes to the science of radiography, allowing technicians to standardize techniques and, thus, reduce the number of retakes.

While the technical aspects of radiology improved, remuneration for technicians themselves did not. X-ray technicians still drew a relatively low salary — a result, perhaps, of the fact that the majority of technicians were women.

But times were changing, and more radiologists were learning to appreciate the value of a well-educated technician. "Diagnostic x-ray technicians are invaluable to the radiologist (and have) become so expert that they are more and more helpful," one radiologist asserted in 1948. "Because of the increasing value of technicians to radiologists, it is believed that they should be appropriately remunerated for their services.... The well-qualified x-ray technician of today is a professional person."

Had credibility for the x-ray technician finally arrived? Not entirely, but some major hurdles were cleared and the Society and Registry had firmly established themselves as powerful forces in determining the future direction of the profession.

The Social Society

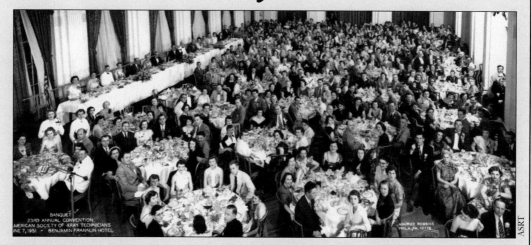

This banquet scene from the 1951 ASXT Annual Conference depicts the grandeur of the era.

In the 1940s and '50s the ASXT was more than just a professional society; it often was a major part of the technician's social life. Chief x-ray technicians stressed the importance of attending annual meetings, families were warmly welcomed, and conference highlights ranged from educational lectures to boating tours. If these meetings were important socially to technicians, they were equally important as business events to manufacturers and distributors of x-ray equipment, who hosted luncheons, banquets, "gadgeteria" sessions and special presentations.

The heyday of the ASXT Annual Conference began in the late 1930s and continued through the 1950s. For the 1937 meeting in Denver, attendees were met at the train station and transported to the hotel in specially decorated cars with huge cardboard skeletons on the front of the radiators. Among the events planned by the Colorado hosts was a trip to Manitou Falls by automobile, highlighted by the escort of the mounted highway patrol, which screamed its way through halted traffic to lead the cavalcade of x-ray technicians to the hotel.

Although security and transportation concerns during World War II forced the ASXT to cancel its 1943, 1944 and 1945 annual conferences, the lack of meetings had no toll on membership figures. The ASXT hosted its first postwar annual meeting in St. Louis, and in deference to the many military-trained technicians instituted what would become the Society's educational hallmark — refresher courses. During the 1946 meeting these courses covered such subjects as atomic theory and electricity; x-ray tubes, machines and radiation; and positioning. The courses were so popular that they became a permanent part of the Annual Conference program, known today as continuing education courses.

The 1949 convention in San Francisco was the Society's 21st, drawing more than 450 attendees. A refresher course presented by John Cahoon, R.T., titled "Formulating X-Ray Exposure Charts and Special Techniques," was filled to capacity and repeated the next year by popular demand. Melvin Aspray, M.D., a Seattle radiologist who attended the San Francisco meeting, was so impressed by the event that he later wrote, "The work and enthusiasm put into a national convention by the technician members is really beyond belief."

In 1951 ASXT President John Cahoon said one of his primary goals for the Society's Annual Conference was to present topnotch educational courses. "Our policy should be to attract refresher-course teachers of the highest caliber and to provide sound scientific programs," he wrote in the September 1950 issue of *The X-Ray Technician*. That policy proved successful as conference attendance continued to grow. Nearly 1,000 people attended the Society's 1952 meeting in Chicago at the Morrison Hotel.

The meetings were popular because they were a perfect blend of business and pleasure; a time to embrace new technologies and renew old friendships. Jack Cullinan, R.T., attended his first ASXT Annual Conference in Philadelphia in 1951. Representatives from x-ray film companies offered Cullinan and other young technicians free rides to the meeting, and Cullinan and his technician wife, Angie, attended the convention's banquet courtesy of an Eastman Kodak representative who "just happened" to have two extra tickets. Recalling that era, Cullinan noted, "Although the main purpose of the Society was education and the promotion of the art and science of radiography, the Society was also an important part of the technician's social life. Families were welcomed and many lasting friendships were made."

Coordinating the annual meeting required the work of dozens of volunteer committee members. Special arrangements always were made to accommodate the many Catholic nuns attending the conference, who were housed at parochial schools in the host city. When such accommodations were unavailable, an entire floor of the conference hotel would be reserved for Sisters only.

Although the Society's annual meeting grew both in size and sophistication through the years, its tradition of education, friendship, progress and unity has endured.

—Paul Young and Ceela McElveny

Chapter Eight

A New Generation of Giants

The profession finally began to realize the fruits of its labors. By the early 1950s the standardization of x-ray technique had raised skills to a new level of expertise, advances in medical technology enhanced the technician's role as a vital member of the health care team, and improvements in radiation protection made the profession more attractive to a younger generation of health care providers. In addition, the ASXT and ARXT had earned a new measure of recognition and respect from the medical community and educational standards were falling into place. There had never been a better time to be an x-ray technician.

Out of this stable environment emerged a new generation of leaders for the profession. Their temperaments ranged from the fiery dedication of Sister Mary Alacoque Anger of St. Louis to the affable, gentlemanly charm of North Carolina's John Cahoon. They were intellectually facile, highly motivated and compassionate, and they all shared a desire to control their own destinies as health care professionals. Never complacent with the status quo, this new generation of giants led the profession into an unprecedented era of expansion.

To recognize the many achievements of these dedicated leaders, ASXT members in

1955 voted to create an additional membership category known as Fellow. In establishing the new category, the Society's Board of Directors noted that those who qualified for the honor "must be not only an excellent technician, but also one who has demonstrated his interest in technicians and their advancement through active educational endeavors, society activities and written papers."

Forty-eight candidates were nominated as charter ASXT Fellows. The 12 who met the rigid requirements were elevated in Louisville, Ky., on June 18, 1956, at the Society's 28th Annual Conference. "It was an inspiring moment to all technicians," noted President Clark Warren, R.T. Included in the prestigious group of charter Fellows were Sister Mary Alacoque Anger, R.T.; John B. Cahoon, R.T.; Erminda Clarke, R.T.; Louis P. Divilio, R.T.; Floyd L. Driver, R.T.; Sister Mary Fides Stolz, R.T.; Alfred B. Greene, R.T.; Edward Gunson, R.T.; Mary Knish Jancosek, R.T.; Sister Mary Beatrice Merrigan, R.T.; Edward M. White, R.T.; and Roy E. Wolcott, R.T.

Reflecting on the significance of their elevation, Clark Warren noted, "This new membership category offers an incentive, a goal for which technicians may strive. We know that by doing so the whole level of technical

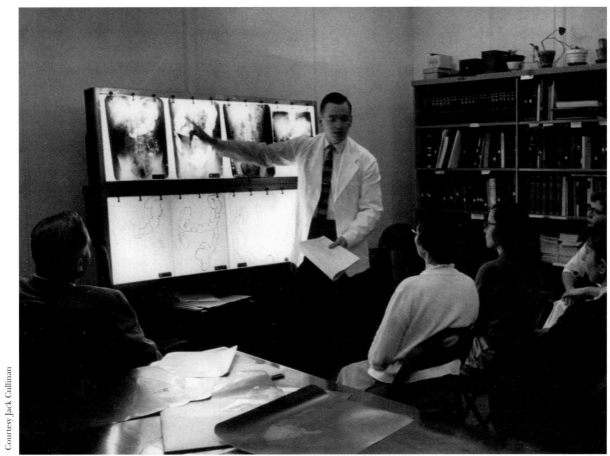

Courtesy Jack Cullinan

1960 - (above) Jack Cullinan lectures to a group of Du Pont employees about radiographic positioning.

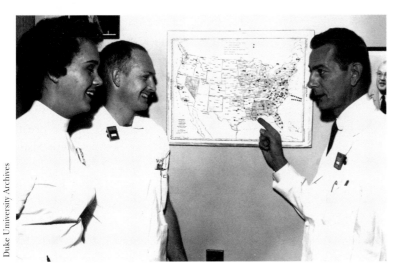

Duke University Archives

1958 - (above) John Cahoon, director of the School of X-Ray Technology at Duke, points out to student technicians the geographical distribution of the school's graduates.

achievement and proficiency will be raised (and) our professional stature will be increased. Those who have given deep thought to this subject feel that the American Society has set up something fine, something which will enrich our future."

The 12 charter Fellows not only represented the Society's greatest achievers, they also accurately reflected the diversity of the profession by 1956. Among them were chief technicians, radiography educators, the executive director of the Registry, three Catholic nuns and two former ASXT presidents. Despite their diversity, however, they shared a common need to help advance their chosen profession. In doing so, they attained an unprecedented measure of self-realization and achievement for themselves and the profession as a whole. To understand these giants is to understand the profession itself.

Sister Mary Alacoque Anger graduated from St. Mary's Infirmary School of Nursing in 1919 and became part of the long tradition of healing the Sisters of St. Mary were known

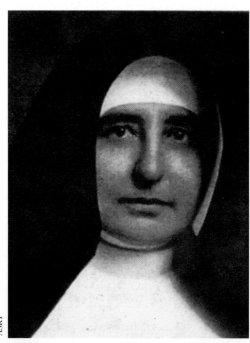

1947 - Sister Mary Alacoque Anger, R.T.

for throughout Missouri. Her interest in x-ray developed during her time as supervisor of the surgical department at the St. Mary's Hospital in Jefferson City. She later transferred to the x-ray program at St. Mary's in St. Louis, where she trained under the supervision of LeRoy Sante, M.D.

In 1928 Sister Mary Alacoque was certified by the American Registry of X-Ray Technicians, and in 1930 she joined the American Society of X-Ray Technicians. In 1931 she was appointed to the ASXT's newly created Council on Education and Registration.

Sister Mary Alacoque's passion and life work revolved around radiologic technology education. She was 30 years ahead of her time in promoting a four-year degree for radiologic technologists. According to one of her former students, Sister Aloysius Marie Borst, Sister Mary Alacoque worked diligently to get a four-year university credit course approved for x-ray technicians.

When St. Louis University's School of Nursing finally approved a bachelor of science degree program in radiologic technology in 1934, Sister Mary Alacoque assisted in its organization. So that students would not have to repeat courses, the Sister insisted that the university recognize and accept credits earned in two-year programs, thus pioneering the only educational program of its kind at the time. She was its first graduate, earning magna cum laude status in 1937 and becoming the first technician in the United States to receive a bachelor of science degree in radiologic technology. Sister Mary Alacoque went on to become program director and assistant professor in the university's radiologic technology program.

In addition to her university work, Sister Mary Alacoque published more than 60 articles and reports in professional journals and prepared scientific exhibits for dozens of local, state and national meetings.

When Black and White Meant More Than X-Rays

For some x-ray technicians in the 1950s and '60s, the job carried far more challenges than merely producing good films. Through the decades, U.S. radiography carried no fewer racial biases than the rest of medicine or popular culture. But at crucial junctures the profession produced a few heroic visionaries.

One such individual was Royce Osborn, R.T., the first African American president of the ASRT. Because of his race, Osborn repeatedly faced rejection for positions he was qualified for and labored for years in segregated hospitals, using outdated or homemade equipment. Despite the obstacles, he produced such good images that white physicians occasionally berated their staffs for not measuring up.

Osborn's career in radiologic technology began by accident — literally. He was helping a friend move a car when another car struck him from behind. Only one of his severely damaged legs was saved; the other was amputated above the knee. The accident occurred during his final year of medical technology training at Massachusetts Memorial Hospital in Boston. He spent six months in and out of the hospital and received many x-rays, becoming friendly with the technologists and impressed by their caring personalities. It was enough to inspire him to pursue a career in x-ray.

His bachelor's degree in biology from Xavier University in New Orleans, combined with his medical technology training, gave him a sound science base that left only the clinical experience to become a radiologic technologist. He soon completed Massachusetts Memorial Hospital's year-

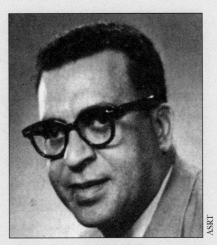

1969 - Royce Osborn, R.T.

long program in radiologic technology, passed the Registry exam and joined the ASXT in 1952. But he couldn't find work in Boston, so he returned to his Southern roots in New Orleans. He worked for three years as a staff technologist at Ft. Polk Army Hospital in New Orleans, where he received a commendation for his research and model of an auxiliary cassette holder. In 1955 he became chief technologist at the Flint-Goodrich Hospital, an all-black hospital in New Orleans, earning $200 a month.

At the time, Osborn recalled, "Emergency rooms had 'Colored' sections, and blacks couldn't be in the same areas as whites." Black physicians in the South were allowed to operate out of "black" hospitals only. Osborn knew several of the technologists at the "white" hospitals and talked to them over the phone, but could not meet with them professionally because their hospitals barred him from participating in any of their educational meetings.

Under such circumstances, Osborn improvised and expanded his own learning. He experimented with new positioning and film techniques, x-raying himself and his family to collect research data for professional papers.

98   *A New Generation of Giants*

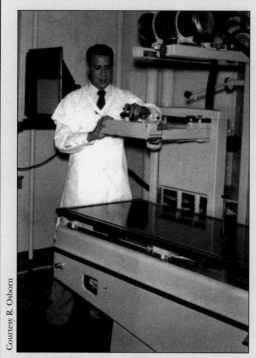

Circa 1958 *– Royce Osborn at work in the
x-ray department of the Flint-Goodrich Hospital.*

At Flint-Goodrich he made his own reci-
procating grid because a new one cost
about $200 — a full month of his salary. The
idea came to him after x-raying a painter's
hand. The spatterings of paint, which contained lead, could be seen on the x-ray.
Osborn made his own grid with a wire brush
and lead-impregnated paint on a square
plate of glass. He suspended the device
above the table with rubber bands.

"The operating room surgeons thought I
was a little crazy, but it worked great and
lasted for years," he said.

His hard work paid off in 1959 when the
ASXT invited him to present a research
paper at the national conference in Denver.
The following year he won a prestigious
research award from an electrical manufacturers association and was elected to the
Society's Public Relations Committee.

Despite his professional successes at the
national level, Osborn lived with prejudice

in the South. Segregation laws in Osborn's
home state prevented his membership in
the Louisiana and New Orleans radiologic
technologist societies, even though he had
been a member of the national Society for
many years.

The issue came to a head in 1966, when
Osborn was nominated for the office of
ASRT vice president. Longtime member
Ted Ott, R.T., recalled that during the 1966
Annual Conference in Boston, attendees
were buzzing with the news that Osborn
had repeatedly been denied membership in
his state society. "I couldn't believe what I
was being told," recalled Ott, who had never
met Osborn before. At the next day's business session, immediately preceding the
election of officers, Ott approached the
microphone.

According to the official minutes of that
meeting, Ott said, "I would like to ask the
Board of Directors of the American Society
of Radiologic Technologists if it is indeed a
fact that active members of this Society have
been repeatedly denied membership in
state societies affiliated with the American
Society of Radiologic Technologists because
of race." When he received an affirmative
answer, Ott continued, "I would therefore
hope that many affiliated societies will prepare amendments to the bylaws for presentation during the next annual meeting of
the American Society of Radiologic Technologists that would require forfeiture of a
charter from any affiliated society that
would prohibit membership because of
race. On this day I am not only sorry, but
ashamed to have to admit membership in
the American Society of Radiologic Technologists!"

When Ott finished his speech, there was
a stunned silence in the auditorium. Then,
suddenly, every ASRT member in atten-

dance rose in a standing ovation. Osborn was elected to the office of vice president, went on to serve two terms as president of the New Orleans society and was elected ASRT president in 1969.

Osborn served his ASRT presidency during a tumultuous year, when the small "social" Society was reshaping itself into a modern medical association. The Society had moved its offices to Chicago, reorganized and hired an executive director. But even with its new professional staff, much of the Society's detail work fell to the president and Board of Directors. Osborn ultimately moved his family to Chicago to be closer to the "home office," where he could more closely follow the major professional issues of the day, including universal position descriptions, federal licensure proposals and minimum performance standards.

At the time, the federal government and certain health care groups were pushing for lower technologist training requirements and safety standards. "I did my (own) letters to the Board," Osborn said. "I had to peck out 10 carbon copies to Board members and affiliates on a beat-up, old typewriter. I was often up until 2 or 3 in the morning, but the work had to get done."

Through it all, Osborn's hallmark was his great attitude and sense of humor. "Once, on my way up to the operating room with the portable unit, my artificial leg got pinned between the elevator doors and the cart," he recalled. "I had to go down to the basement to fix it. Meanwhile, the surgeon was asking where I was, and somebody told him that I broke my leg and had gone to the basement to fix it. He didn't know I had a prosthesis and couldn't figure out why I had gone to the basement to get it fixed!"

—*Barbara Pongracz-Bartha*

Editor's Note: In June 1995 Royce Osborn was diagnosed with terminal cancer. He was impressed with the skill and professionalism of the magnetic resonance and nuclear medicine technologists during his diagnostic tests.

"I feel positive that we have good people in the profession. The profession is in good hands. I am very proud to be a radiologic technologist," he said.

She spent 40 years at St. Louis University and retired as director of the School of Radiologic Technology in June 1969. She'd just finished clearing out her office and had gone to the kitchen for a cup of soup when she collapsed and died, just minutes after starting her official retirement.

The Sisters of St. Mary chronicle Sister Mary Alacoque as "frank and humorous, simple and candid. Her direct approach often startled people and her natural aggressiveness frequently rubbed them the wrong way. But there were few who failed to recognize that she possessed a heart of gold, ready to give of itself without stint or measure."

Sister Alacoque was one of many who dedicated their lives to the education of x-ray technicians. John B. Cahoon Jr., R.T., was another.

Cahoon was one of the most highly respected educators and leaders the profession ever produced. He rose from a "soda jerk" at a Duke University malt shop in Durham, N.C., to authoring a landmark textbook, chairing the Duke University School of Medicine X-Ray Program, helping form the North Carolina affiliate society, being elected ASXT president in 1950-51, serving as a trustee on the Registry Board from 1954 to 1959, and being named a charter Fellow of the ASXT in 1956.

Cahoon was a perfectionist who pursued excellence in everything, down to the formal manner of his speech and his dapper clothes. He chose education as the mechanism

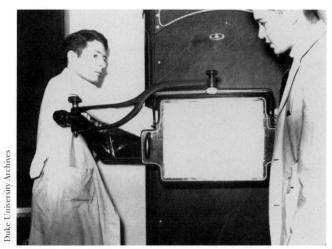

***1938** - John Cahoon (left) during his student days at Duke University.*

through which he pursued perfection, demanding excellence from his students and colleagues alike. Cynthia Easterling, R.T., who was elevated to ASRT Fellow in 1980 and served as Society president in 1981, was one of Cahoon's students at Duke. Recalling her classes with the professor, she said, "He was dignified, an impeccable dresser, confident in manner and almost giant-like to some of us. Sitting in his classroom was often thrilling but frightening, because he was a perfectionist and demanded perfection." Easterling described how Cahoon would "inspect" his students, explaining, "We would sit up straight. We'd take one last glance at our white clinic shoes, hoping they would be unscuffed. His eyes would briefly but adeptly scan students, and he could spot a scuff from eight rows back or spy uncombed hair and counter with, 'Drop by my office and I'll show you what a comb is.' His classes were precise, never canceled, and at times almost heart-failing."

Whether lecturing before a classroom full of students or an auditorium full of peers, Cahoon was effortlessly comfortable at the podium, displaying elements of the showman and the comedian. Many described him as an icon for the profession, but there were detrac-

tors who characterized Cahoon as "a bad guy with a lot of good publicity" who could carry hefty grudges.

Cahoon's entry into the profession was unorthodox. Longtime friend Frances Apple, R.T.(R), who followed Cahoon at Duke, said radiology professor R.J. Reeves, M.D., "discovered" Cahoon in the soda shop and interested him in x-ray. He graduated in x-ray technology from Duke University School of Medicine in 1940 and was certified by the Registry that same year. He was appointed chief x-ray technician at Duke University Hospital in 1942 and hired by the hospital as an instructor in x-ray technology in 1943.

After joining the national Society in 1941, Cahoon became fanatical in his advocacy of the ASXT, stressing the importance of attending even the sometimes lengthy business sessions at the Society's conferences. Any student of Cahoon's who did not attend these meetings could expect Cahoon "to come looking for you," Frances Apple recalls. Apple herself was elevated to a Fellow in the Society in 1987.

Despite what she characterized as the complexity and often maddening aspects of his personality, Apple acknowledged, "John Cahoon is the single person who made me into the technologist that I am today. He really did give me so much."

A very direct writer, Cahoon penned a wonderfully concise and hugely significant textbook titled *Formulating X-Ray Technic*, published in 1948. The Cahoon book was the first comprehensive text on radiographic technique since Ed Jerman's *Modern X-Ray Technic*, published nearly 20 years earlier. It was a lifesaver for hundreds of technicians-in-training and became the standard educational text for many x-ray programs.

Cahoon was revered for his professionalism and vast knowledge of the practice. He taught his students these lessons and, perhaps more importantly, instilled in them the value of membership in the national Society as a way to achieve peer respect and build personal self-esteem — something that still was lacking among many technicians. He even taught his young protégés how to act in social and professional situations.

Perhaps because of his influence on the high-profile ASXT Education Committee, on which he served as chairman in 1949, Cahoon frequently was able to lure big names in the profession for the North Carolina Society meetings, including Alfred B. Greene, who by that point was a legend in radiography.

Cahoon delivered the Ed Jerman Memorial Lecture at the 1960 ASXT Annual Conference. His topic was "Radiographic Technique — Its Origin, Concept, Practical Application and Evaluation of Radiation Dosage," and he drew a full house. The Jerman Memorial Lecture had been created in 1946 to honor scholarship within the Society. Its goal was to recognize Society members who emulated Jerman's dedication to study and research. When Cahoon died in December 1973, he was a member of the Society's Committee on Memorial Lectures. In 1974 his colleagues on that committee asked the Society to establish a John B. Cahoon Memorial Lecture that would alternate every other year with the Jerman Lecture.

The first Cahoon Memorial Lecture was delivered in 1978 by his former Duke student Cynthia Easterling. The subject of her lecture was John Cahoon himself. She said of her teacher, "After all is said and done, there is no way that anyone could say that the professor was not a giant. He had the knack for motivating people. To some it was out of fear; to others it was out of respect. He left some awfully big shoes to fill when death called him prematurely."

Two of John Cahoon's best professional friends were themselves giants in the profession — Bill Conklin, R.T., who was elevated to

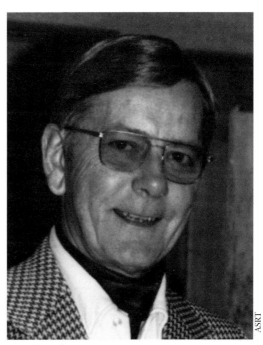

Circa 1970 - *John B. Cahoon Jr., R.T.*

ASXT Fellow in 1962, and John (Jack) Cullinan, R.T., who was elevated to Fellow in 1968. During the 1950s and '60s, the trio of Cahoon, Conklin and Cullinan gained great notoriety as "The Three C's Traveling Lecture Show," journeying from state to state to teach fellow technicians.

"Cahoon talked about technique, Cullinan talked about special procedures and I discussed positioning," Conklin explained. They were highly respected lecturers on the affiliate-conference circuit, but they were not necessarily somber academics. "It wasn't out of character for practical jokes to be played," Conklin recalled. "Sometimes I'd mess up Cahoon's illuminators so they'd be out of position." But the three men remained the best of friends throughout their careers.

Like many x-ray technicians of the era, Bill Conklin's entrance into the profession was unplanned. He was sitting in a Knights of Columbus Hall in 1949, contemplating what to do with his life after the Marines. His father casually mentioned an on-the-job opening in

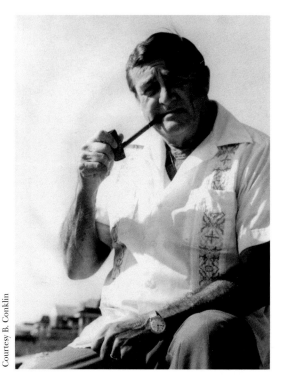

Courtesy B. Conklin

1982 - Bill Conklin, R.T.

the x-ray department at Roper Hospital in Charleston, S.C., where Conklin could work on patients during the day and take classes at night. Conklin thought this sounded like an interesting opportunity and decided to investigate. Four decades later, Conklin had educated hundreds of x-ray students and still was lecturing occasionally.

One of Conklin's first jobs in radiography was at St. Elizabeth's Mental Hospital in Washington, D.C., where "the x-ray department looked like Roentgen had just left the lab." Most of the staff was male because of the physical strength often required to restrain patients. "While I was there," Conklin recalled, "I x-rayed the American poet Ezra Pound, who said that he was at St. Elizabeth's to avoid going to jail." Pound was to be tried on charges of treason following World War II. "Many of the patients were sane but acted crazy to avoid jail," Conklin said.

In 1956 Conklin moved to Duvall Medical Center, a 300-bed facility in Jacksonville, Fla.,

where he served as chief technologist. But eventually he returned to his beloved Carolinas and, appropriately enough, took a position at the Orangeburg Cahoon Memorial Hospital in Orangeburg, S.C. — named after his old friend and lecture companion, John Cahoon.

Conklin went on to make quite a name for himself in radiographic art by x-raying unusual shapes such as conch shells. Two books featuring his shell radiographs have been published.

Many other deserving individuals rose to leadership positions in the Society through hard work and dedication. Their tales of professional and personal achievement are inspirational to all technologists.

One of the Society's grand ladies and strongest promoters was Margaret Hoing, R.T. Born in 1881, Hoing entered nurses' training at the age of 31 at Frances E. Willard National Temperance Hospital in Chicago. After becoming a registered nurse in 1919, her interests were directed toward radiologic technology by Benjamin H. Orndoff, M.D., the radiologist who organized the radiology department at Loyola University School of Medicine and was a founder of the American College of Radiology. Hoing became registered as an x-ray technician in 1923, immediately joined the American Society of X-Ray Technicians and became close friends with Ed Jerman, the man whose life she would later chronicle.

The depth and duration of Hoing's involvement with the Society was unsurpassed. She attended every Annual Conference of the Society from 1923 to 1966 and served on every ASXT committee. A great motivator, especially when it came to recruiting new members to the Society, she was elected ASXT president in 1931 and awarded lifetime membership in 1940.

In 1946, Hoing was appointed the Society's

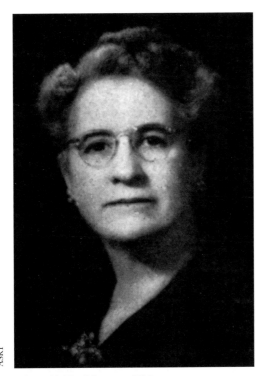

Circa 1945 - Margaret Hoing

first historian — a duty she described as "the greatest that I have ever assumed since the organization of the Society." During the next several years, she took on the enormous task of writing the first formal history of the national Society and its founders, painstakingly chronicling every Annual Conference and Board of Directors meeting.

Her commitment to the profession kept Hoing working as an x-ray technician well into her 80s, working for Dr. Orndoff in Chicago from 1923 until he retired in 1968. Known as a serious thinker, she occasionally showed a lighter side. A favorite hobby of hers was vacationing in different parts of the United States, investigating old cemeteries. On one occasion traveling through New England, she stopped at Franklin D. Roosevelt's grave "just to make sure he was in it."

Hoing died on Feb. 12, 1978, at the age of 96.

One of Hoing's dearest friends was Virginia Milligan, R.T., who was active in the profession for nearly three decades before

ascending to the Society presidency in 1975. She started out pursuing a nursing career, but in 1944 she worked briefly in the radiology department of St. Anne's Hospital in Chicago and decided to switch to the hospital's two-year program in radiologic technology.

"Most of the classes were hit-and-miss," she said, noting that many of the courses were really designed for nurses. So she eventually began individual study and clinical learning under the supervision of St. Anne's nuns and a radiologist. Three nights a week, four hours per night, she studied physics and the principles of x-ray technique at the General Electric Building in downtown Chicago. Students received a $50 stipend monthly, and Milligan earned an additional $25 per month for transcription work.

When she entered the profession in the late 1940s, "only the radiologists were issued lead aprons," Milligan recalled. The importance of safety for technicians wasn't really stressed. "For chest x-rays, two technologists on each side of the patient would hold up the film," she said. "Later, when safety became a concern, we built a chest holder for the film and the patient."

Milligan also recalled how vital technicians were to non-radiologists in the hospital. "In the late '40s and early '50s, we did x-ray exams for all the doctors, not just the radiologists," she explained. "But when these doctors read the films, most didn't know what to look for. I'd help them interpret the films, but in a very subtle way. For example, I'd point to a significant area on the film and ask, 'What do you suppose that means?'"

During the course of the next 45 years, Milligan played a variety of important roles within the national Society. In particular, she remembers with fondness her duties as general chairman for the ASRT International Convention held in Chicago in 1965, a conjoint meeting of the American and Canadian societies. "I was very concerned that everything go well, especially for the Canadians," Milligan said. She and the props chairman set up the room for the ASRT business meeting and positioned the U.S. and Canadian flags at the doors. Milligan told the props chairman not to let anyone touch the flags, then left to take care of other business.

"Shortly before the meeting, I was approached by the hotel manager and one of the Canadians," Milligan recalled. "Apparently, there was only one Canadian flag in the entire hotel and they needed it for the Canadian society meetings, but the props chairman wouldn't let them have it. Immediately after our business meeting, I grabbed the flag and ran it over to the Canadian meeting. I spent the entire rest of the convention running back and forth with that flag!"

Such acts of dedication were typical of Society members. Milligan retired in 1991 from her position as director of the St. Joseph Hospital School of Radiologic Technology in Phoenix, Ariz.

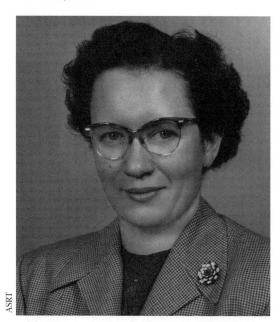

Ruth Jaffke contributed many articles to the Society journal in the 1950s and '60s. She was elevated to Fellow in 1971.

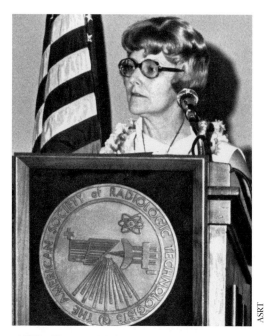

1975 *- Virginia Milligan became ASRT president.*

Unlike so many of her colleagues who worked in hospitals, Ruth Jaffke, R.T., spent her career with the People's Gas Company in Chicago. But what a place to work! The gas company had its own industrial medical department staffed with six physicians and four nurses. It served 15,000 employees, providing x-ray, lab work, blood studies, EKGs and other health care services.

Jaffke developed at least two new radiographic procedures as a practicing technician. The first was a tissue measurement technique that was later addressed in a chapter of John Cahoon's book. The second innovation resulted in a classic research paper titled "Why the Additional View." Jaffke was elevated to Fellow in the Society in 1971.

The editor of Jaffke's many technical papers in *The X-Ray Technician* was Jean Inglis Widger, R.T. No list of giants of the profession would be complete without Widger's inclusion. The daughter of an English professor who stressed the best in spoken and written language, Widger was hired for her first job, as a reporter for her hometown newspaper, while still in high school. She earned 10 cents an inch for everything she wrote that was printed.

After graduating from the University of Illinois with a baccalaureate degree in bacteriology and taking courses in journalism at the University of Michigan, Widger directed her interests toward a career in radiologic technology. She became an ASXT member in 1949 and immediately was appointed to the Society's publication committee.

Widger worked as an x-ray technician in Illinois and Michigan before moving into the world of academia, joining Wayne State University in Detroit as an administrative assistant in 1958 and taking over the university's graduate school journal. Although no longer working in the profession, Widger maintained her Registry certification and Society membership and always considered herself to be an x-ray technician.

In January 1956 Widger was named editor of the ASXT journal, *The X-Ray Technician*. It was a task to which she devoted the next quarter century of her life. Under Widger's expert guidance, the journal's name was changed to *Radiologic Technology* in 1963 and grew into a highly respected and internationally acclaimed bimonthly, publishing some of the top research in the profession.

During her long tenure as editor of the journal, Widger transformed many reticent technicians into published authors. "Jean Widger gave me tons of encouragement and support when I really needed it," recalled Jack Cullinan, who published several technical articles in the Society journal during the 1960s and '70s. "She was a mentor to many fledgling writers in the profession. If she said you could do it, you believed you could do it."

When Widger died in 1980, she was mourned throughout the professional community. In her memory, the Society created

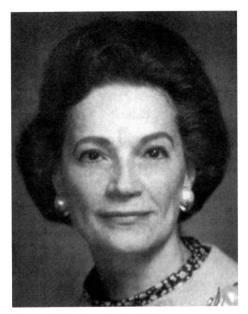

Circa 1970 - Jean Inglis Widger

the Jean I. Widger Distinguished Author Award, presented annually to the author or authors of the best peer-reviewed manuscript published in the Society's journal.

Widger delivered the Jerman Memorial Lecture in 1969, becoming only the sixth woman out of 24 individuals to receive the honor. During her lecture, she briefly discussed the giants of the profession's past. Each of these giants, she explained, "possessed a drive, a dedication, a sincere concern for his chosen field. Each has strived to make the most of his potential. Each has spent his personal life in the pursuit of excellence. Not only was each of these individuals concerned with the development of his own potential, but each was dedicated to the establishment of standards for others — for the highest possible development of talent in a field which is challenging, which is dedicated to bringing to humanity the highest degree of excellence in the diagnosis and treatment of human ills."

Today's technologists are the inheritors of that tradition of excellence.

Mr. and Mrs. X-Ray

If you want to know how tomography evolved or what technologists thought of physicians in the 1950s or why thermography never caught on, all you need to do is spend a little time with Jack and Angie Cullinan.

The Cullinans know the profession's history because they helped write so much of it.

Between them, Jack Cullinan, R.T., and Angie Cullinan, R.T., devoted nearly 90 years to the radiologic sciences. They were technologists, administrators, educators and authors; they served as JRCERT site visitors, ARRT item writers and local society presidents; they worked in clinical research, the commerical arena and the military.

And along the way, the Cullinans influenced an entire generation of technologists. Jack Cullinan's *Illustrated Guide to X-Ray Technics* was required reading in many educational programs throughout the 1970s, and Angie Cullinan's groundbreaking work in the mid-1960s led to the development of screen-film mammography.

Through it all, the Cullinans' goal was to inspire other technologists to achieve successes even greater than their own. "Behind everything we did was an overwhelming need to teach others how to do it even better," explained Jack.

Perhaps radiologic technology became such a major part of the Cullinans' lives because the x-ray brought them together in the first place. Jack and Angie met on Oct. 17, 1950, at an educational meeting sponsored by District 7 of the Pennsylvania Society of X-Ray Technicians.

At the time, Angie was a radiography student at Mercy Hospital in Wilkes-Barre, Pa. Her education in x-ray was far from formal; she didn't even have a textbook. "I just sat across the desk from the nun in charge of the x-ray department, Sister Mary Frances, and she would talk about kVp or explain how to perform a particular procedure."

While Angie was studying in Wilkes-Barre, Jack was working as an orderly at Hazleton State Hospital in Hazleton, Pa., where he became fascinated with the state-of-the-art technology in the radiology department. The hospital's radiography program followed the old medical preceptorship of "See one, do one, teach one." Explained Jack, "You watched an exam being performed and the next day you performed it yourself and the day after that you taught another student how to do it."

The Cullinans both recall some unusual methods of radiation protection during their student days. Angie was required to sit under an ultraviolet light twice a week to protect herself from x-rays. She'd wind up getting a dreadful sunburn.

Some of the ideas about radiation protection seem odd now, agreed Jack. "I was required to eat liver once a week because they thought it would protect us from ane-

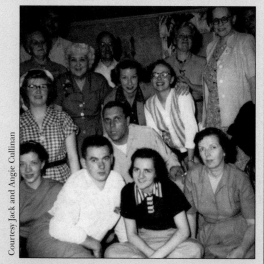

Courtesy Jack and Angie Cullinan

Jack and Angie (front row, center) at a 1951 meeting of District 7 of the Pennsylvania Society of X-Ray Technicians.

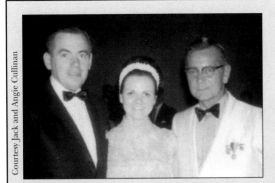

Jack and Angie Cullinan with John Cahoon at the 1969 ASRT meeting in Atlanta.

mia. The hospital performed blood counts on all the technicians once a month. If your hemoglobin was low, they took you out of the x-ray department for a while. We wore lead gloves and aprons, but we didn't wear badges." Jack never even saw a badge until 1955, after he'd been working in x-ray more than five years.

"There just wasn't as much concern as maybe there should have been," he acknowledged. "This was 50 years after Roentgen discovered the x-ray and there'd been all these people who'd lost fingers and limbs to radiation, yet the attitude was that if someone had to hold a baby who needed an x-ray, you'd just go in there and hold the baby."

Angie became registered in November 1951, when she was 18. Jack sat for the Registry exam a year later. Both joined the ASXT immediately after becoming registered.

When Jack and Angie married on Oct. 3, 1953, they both worked at hospitals in the Wilkes-Barre area. "It was a much more innocent time," remembered Angie, "and as technicians we were taught to respect the authority of the physician. You actually stood up whenever one of them entered the room. But it was a two-way street. You respected them, and they trusted you."

Jack agreed. "We were in complete awe of the physicians, but we knew they were human too. Sometimes the young interns would beg the technicians to read an x-ray for them because they had so little experience and didn't know what they were looking at. Of course, we weren't allowed to read the x-rays, so we had to dance around the subject. We'd point out an area and ask, 'What do you think this could be? Could it be a fracture?' Or we'd see an x-ray of a collapsed lung and the intern would come in and say everything looked fine. That was when we had to step in and say, 'Oh, doctor, what is this long gray line on the side over here? Is that the lung pulling away?' We had to pretend we didn't know what it was."

The Cullinans' first two daughters, Jeanne and Patty, were born in 1954 and 1955 and Angie left the profession temporarily to stay home and raise them. Then, in 1955, Jack enlisted in the Naval Reserves and was sent to the U.S. Naval Hospital in Philadelphia. Jack figured the Navy would have the latest technology, and he was right.

Following his two-year stint in the Navy, Jack obtained a $100-per-week position as chief technologist at the Albert Einstein Medical Center in Philadelphia, which had one of the first cardiopulmonary labs in the area and one of the first Kodak X-Omat automatic processors in the United States.

The Cullinan family grew with the arrival of Diane in 1959 and Terry in 1961. When their youngest daughter was 5, Angie went back to work full-time, joining Jack at Albert Einstein Medical Center as supervisor of the mammography and thermography departments. Because the mammographic examinations of that era delivered a high radiation dose, many hospitals used thermography to screen women for suspected tumors before subjecting them to a mammogram.

At that time, many physicians did not believe in the effectiveness of mammograms. But Angie began working with Jacob Gershon-Cohen, M.D., the premier mammography expert in the country, on a breast cancer detection project. As a member of Gershon-Cohen's team, she helped screen hundreds of women who had no exhibited symptoms of breast cancer. The research team discovered more than 30 unsuspected carcinomas, thus establishing mammography as an accurate tool for breast cancer detection.

Although the project proved that mammograms were effective, there was still the question of safety. At the time, mammographic exposures were long because they required industrial-type film. Angie began working with physicians Harold Isard, Bernard Ostram and Warren Becker to uncover a way to produce a high quality image while delivering the lowest possible dose to the patient. Angie's job was to figure out the technical aspects. She experimented for more than a year with different screen and film combinations to produce the lowest dose possible.

Her results were presented to DuPont, which used them to develop a screen-film system that later came to be known as the DuPont Lo-Dose system. In 1972, when DuPont was ready to introduce the product commercially, it asked Angie to pose as the technologist in the advertisements.

The introduction of screen-film systems was the turning point for mammography. As a result of the DuPont screen-film technique, total dose to the patient was reduced 10 to 20 times and physicians began recommending that at-risk women undergo annual mammographic screenings. By 1975 additional advances in screen-film combinations had halved the exposure of the first mammographic systems.

By this time, radiography wasn't just Jack and Angie's livelihood; it was their lives. They were lecturing, writing articles and attending every local society meeting as well as many of the national meetings. The Cullinans' four daughters enjoyed their parents' involvement in the profession, often accompanying them to conferences. Usually, at least one of them was in the audience while their parents lectured on stage.

Jack recalled one presentation when he posed a question about grids that no one in the audience could answer. Frustrated, he lectured for 20 more minutes on the topic and then asked the question again. Still no response. Finally, a small voice from the back of the room called out the correct answer. "Who said that?" Jack called. "It was me, daddy," responded 12-year-old Patty from the last row.

Jack's popularity as a lecturer was based on his easygoing presentation style, leading

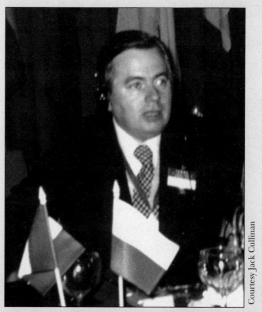

Jack Cullinan lectured at the 1973 International Society of Radiographers and Radiological Technologists meeting in Madrid.

Courtesy Jack Cullinan

some to call him the country's only "stand-up radiographer." But as he began speaking at more and more meetings during the late 1960s, Jack realized that very few people really understood x-ray technique. That's when he decided to write a book.

Jack struggled with how to present the material and even enrolled in a writing course, all to no avail. Finally, Angie rescued him. She told him to sit down at the kitchen table and talk to her, one technologist to another. They tape-recorded their conversations, which became the manuscript for the book.

Published in 1972 by J.B. Lippincott, Jack Cullinan's *Illustrated Guide to X-Ray Technics* was an instant success. Lippincott sold several thousand copies before the book was even printed, based on the advertising alone, because everyone was so hungry for a new text on x-ray technique.

The book went on to become the standard radiography text for many x-ray programs, educating an entire generation of students. When the second edition was published in 1980, Angie joined her husband as coauthor and the Cullinans gained celebrity status at student meetings. "I remember one meeting where we spent two hours autographing books," said Jack. "Then when we tried to leave, some kids actually chased after our car until we stopped and got out to sign more books. It was then that we realized we were teaching thousands of people whom we'd never even met."

In 1974 Jack was offered what he still calls his "dream job" — a chance to join Eastman Kodak in Rochester, N.Y., as the company's clinical and technical support director. It was the job that one of his idols, Arthur Fuchs, held years before.

While employed by Kodak, Jack spoke at more than 100 state and local technician programs annually. He also traveled extensively overseas, particularly in Latin America and the Pacific Rim, educating radiographers around the world about the clinical applications of Kodak products.

Jack and Angie's dedication to the profession did not go unrewarded. Jack was elevated to ASRT Fellow, the Society's highest honor, in 1968. At that time, the Society required 75 points to be eligible for Fellow status; Jack had nearly 300. One of Jack's heroes, John Cahoon, sponsored his elevation to Fellow. Ten years later, Angie was sponsored for ASRT Fellow by her own hero — Jack himself — making the Cullinans the only ASRT Fellows who are married to each other.

Looking back on their long careers, the Cullinans agree that the greatest reward was the chance they had to educate others. "What good is knowledge if you don't share it?" asked Jack. "Our generation of technologists helped make the rules, and Angie and I felt an obligation to pass those rules on to others. We always believed we were educators who happened to work for a hospital or happened to work for Kodak. First and foremost, we were teachers."

It's no surprise, then, that the dedication of one of the many books the Cullinans wrote together reads, "To all who are willing to share what they know." It's the philosophy they lived by throughout their careers.

— *Ceela McElveny*

Chapter Nine

Technician Becomes Technologist

Revolution was a theme throughout America during the decade between 1964 and 1974 as cultural shifts forced the country to re-evaluate almost every aspect of American society. The civil rights movement, the Vietnam War, women's demands for equality in the workplace, educational reforms and an explosion of new technology combined to make the decade one of the most turbulent in U.S. history. Americans walked on the moon and 18-year-olds won the right to vote in national elections; thousands marched on the Washington Mall and in the streets of Chicago while thousands more fought in the jungles of southeast Asia.

Although far less dramatic than the social and political changes occurring all around it, the profession of radiologic technology underwent a revolution of its own. During this decisive decade in the profession's history, the American Society of X-Ray Technicians succeeded in elevating educational standards for technologists, reversed its long-held opposition to licensure and was forced to become involved in socioeconomic issues for the first time.

One of the first signs of the changing times came in 1964, when the technologists' professional society changed its name from the American Society of X-Ray Technicians to the American Society of Radiologic Technologists. The Society's name change was spurred by the Registry. In 1962 members of the ARXT Board of Trustees proposed changing the Registry's name to the American Registry of Radiologic Technologists. The board members believed the term "x-ray technician" was limiting, especially in light of the fact that the Registry was preparing to implement certification exams in nuclear medicine and radiation therapy. The Registry began using its new name in mid-1963, and the first certification exam in nuclear medicine, or "isotope technology," took place during November of that year. The first radiation therapy certification exam was administered in November 1964. For the first time in history, radiologic technologists could become multicredentialed.

Because certification by the Registry was prerequisite to membership in the Society, the ASXT Board of Directors decided to change the name of their organization as well. The Society was representing more and more radiation therapists and nuclear medicine technologists, so the term "x-ray technician" no longer accurately reflected the membership. The name change also reinforced a fine semantic distinction between technician — a term the Society believed

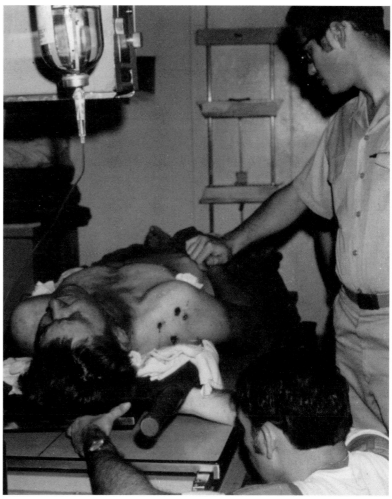

1971 - Examining a wounded soldier with an overhead x-ray unit in the radiology department aboard the U.S.S. Sanctuary, *a Navy hospital ship deployed in Vietnam.*

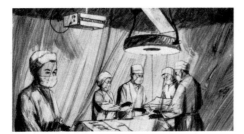

Now you can be in two (or more) places at once

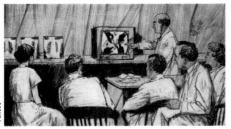

with a Westinghouse closed circuit TV monitoring system

1964 - As this Westinghouse ad for a closed-circuit television system shows, technology began to enter hospitals like never before. Television systems allowed physicians to view x-ray films on monitors, observe surgical operations and watch patients during radiation therapy treatments.

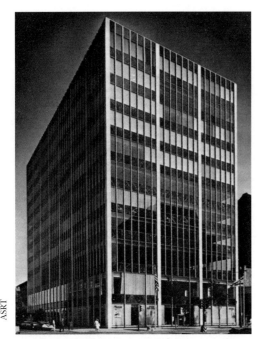

1968 - The ASRT relocated from Fond du Lac, Wis., to Chicago. Its first office in the Windy City was in the John Blair Building at 645 North Michigan Avenue.

implied a worker with minimal on-the-job training — and technologist, a highly skilled, well-educated professional. The change became official following the Society's 1964 Annual Conference.

Other changes were shaping the Registry, the Society and the profession as a whole. After more than 32 years in the Registry office, Alfred Greene retired from his position as executive director in 1966. The ARRT reins were handed over to Roland McGowan, R.T., who resigned from his post as chairman of the ASRT Board to take the position. The ASRT in 1968 relocated its offices from Fond du Lac, Wis., to Chicago and hired its first executive director, Robert C. Best. The ASRT's first director of education, Robert L. Coyle, R.T., was hired shortly afterward.

Technology continued to fuel almost every facet of the profession. Computed tomography came into use in the early 1970s, providing a hundred-fold increase in the amount of

information compared to conventional x-ray techniques. The development of rare-earth imaging systems in the 1970s offered higher speed so technologists could shorten exposure times and, thus, reduce patient dosage. Once-exotic procedures such as mammography and sonography became commonplace and computer-driven systems were installed in more and more radiology departments. The task of turning energy into images was becoming increasingly sophisticated.

As John Cahoon noted in his 1970 lecture at the annual meeting of the North Carolina Society of Radiologic Technologists, "The simple triad of tube, patient and film of former years has given way to complications of image amplification and optics, solid-state locked-in television systems, special cine radiography, automatic processing, 70 and 90 mm serialography, three-phase generators, color subtraction techniques, millisecond timing, and special programming equipment using punch card systems and vacuum cassettes for better detail and duplication of technique." Seemingly overnight, radiology had progressed from the use of a simple glass tube and photographic plate to electronic marvels capable of producing, transmitting and recording x-ray images.

And, as always, the brunt of this explosion in technology was borne by technologists. Radiology could not progress without them.

By the mid-1960s, registered radiologic technologists had a knowledge of radiation that just a few decades earlier was achieved by only a few college professors. The demand for qualified technologists reached a new apex. Between 1947 and 1967, the number of hospital beds in the United States increased by only 20 percent, but the number of x-ray examinations quadrupled. In 1965 the Surgeon General's National Advisory Committee on Radiation estimated that the diagnostic radiology load would continue to increase at a rate of more than 7 percent annually, the radiation therapy load would rise at least 2 percent per year and the demand for nuclear medicine procedures would grow 15 percent annually.

But technological advances weren't the only factors increasing the radiology department's patient load. President Lyndon B. Johnson signed the Medicare Act into law on July 30, 1965, expanding health services to a large new segment of the U.S. population. The profession again found itself facing a serious personnel shortage and in desperate need of new recruits.

The personnel shortage was blamed on low salaries, low status and a lack of opportunity for advancement. At the 1966 National Conference on X-Ray Technician Training, sponsored by the U.S. Public Health Service's Division of Radiological Health, attendees discussed ways to alleviate these conditions. They proposed better educational programs, more scholarships, more rigid inspection of schools, development of continuing education programs and — most significantly — the establishment of minimum nationwide standards to prevent unqualified technologists from operating medical x-ray equipment.

The Society had long opposed such standards, even adopting a policy statement in 1965 stating its belief that "licensure of radiologic technologists by state governments will hinder, rather than help, the achievement of our goal of improved levels of performance in radiologic technology."

Puerto Rico began licensing radiologic technologists in 1963, but it was not until the New York state legislature enacted a licensure law in 1965 that the ASRT began to worry. Confirming the Society's worst fears, the New York law did not include radiation therapists or nuclear medicine technologists and was not the equivalent of the minimum educational standards espoused by the ASRT and the Registry. Other states seemed ready to follow suit, and the Society was concerned that each of the 50 states would devise its own licensure bill, many of which could have lower educational standards than those the profession had struggled to establish nationally.

Such action would destroy years of effort to raise technologists' education standards. At the time, the profession finally was achieving success in eliminating many of the "diploma mills" that churned out x-ray technologists who had little formal training. This latest battle to raise educational standards began in 1959, when the ASRT, Registry and ACR Commission on Technologist Affairs recommended that educational programs for radiologic technologists be two years in length. The recommendation was approved by the ACR Board of Chancellors in early 1960 and ratified by the AMA House of Delegates later that year. Beginning in July 1962, radiologic technology schools had to offer a minimum of 24 months training to receive approval from the AMA Council on Medical Education.

During the next several years, schools revised their curricula to meet the two-year

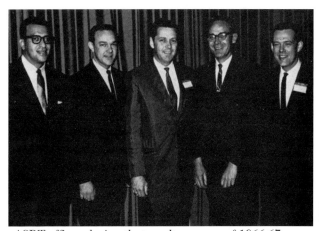

ASRT officers during the tumultuous year of 1966-67 were (left to right) Royce Osborn, secretary-treasurer; David Williams, second vice president; Ralph Coates, first vice president; Neil Lyons, president-elect; and Leslie Wilson, president. Wilson held the office of ASRT president twice, serving again in 1970-71.

Vietnam Remembered

It didn't matter whether they worked out of Army MASH units in the field or Navy hospital ships stationed off the coast; whether they volunteered for their assignment or were drafted; whether they were educated in two-year programs in the states or trained practically overnight by the military. All that mattered was that they helped save lives during one of the most brutal wars in American history.

American radiologic technologists began arriving in Vietnam as early as 1955, when

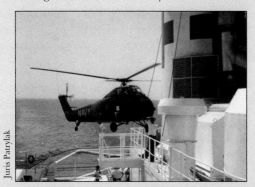

A medical evacuation helicopter comes in for a landing on the U.S.S. Sanctuary.

the United States first sent medical personnel, engineers and agriculture experts to shore up the southern part of the country. South Vietnam recently had been separated at the 17th parallel from its communist neighbor to the north. At the time, many U.S. politicians believed the country would be reunified within only a few years. But in the late 1950s North Vietnam began launching armed assaults on the south, and as the 1960s dawned the U.S. Public Health Service was issuing calls for additional medical personnel to staff provincial hospitals in South Vietnam.

From those early voluntary efforts, U.S. involvement in Vietnam rapidly escalated. Military troops were deployed in ever-

increasing numbers. In 1966 U.S. troop strength in Vietnam numbered 250,000. By 1969 the figure swelled to half a million. Providing medical assistance to the U.S. military and to South Vietnamese civilians became an enormous task.

The radiologic technologists stationed at the Army field hospitals and Navy hospital ships during the Vietnam War treated injuries unlike any they'd ever witnessed at home. The patients they examined were the victims of snipers' bullets, mortar attacks and napalm burns. Among the worst injuries were those caused by booby traps, such as hidden mines in rice paddies and giant spikes concealed along the paths and roadways.

Technologists aboard the two Navy hospital ships, the *U.S.S. Repose* and *U.S.S. Sanctuary*, saw the mind-numbing carnage every day.

The *Repose* arrived at Chu Lai, Vietnam, in early 1966. Sailing up and down the coast between Da Nang and the demilitarized

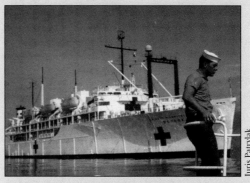

The Navy hospital ship U.S.S. Repose *in Da Nang harbor, 1971.*

zone, the ship's crew treated military and civilian casualties airlifted from the field by medical evacuation helicopters. Only one year after its arrival in Vietnam, the *Repose* saw its 3,000th consecutive helicopter landing.

To share the overwhelming workload,

the *Sanctuary* joined the *Repose* in Vietnam in April 1967. As the war escalated, so did the casualty load. By October 1969 more than 22,000 patients had been treated on the *Repose*, with a slightly smaller total on the *Sanctuary*.

Juris Patrylak, R.T., served on the *U.S.S. Sanctuary* for nearly a year as a diagnostic and special procedures technologist. After graduating from the radiologic technology program at Yale-New Haven Hospital in 1966 and becoming certified by the Registry, Patrylak enlisted in the Navy and was assigned to Portsmouth Naval Hospital in Portsmouth, N.H., in 1968. In 1970 he was reassigned to the radiology department aboard the *Sanctuary* as a hospital corpsman, 2nd class petty officer.

"The ship had a well-equipped radiology department," recalled Patrylak. "It had three radiographic rooms, a darkroom with an automatic processor, an area for viewing radiographs and offices for the radiologists. We had tomography and fluoroscopy capabilities and two General Electric units with image intensifiers." Three ARRT-registered radiologic technologists and two unregistered technicians worked in the department.

"When I first arrived," Patrylak said, "the chief technologist asked how quickly I could do a whole body x-ray. I said it would probably take 30 or 40 minutes. He laughed and told me I'd have to learn to do it in less than 10." The head-to-toe exams were necessary to locate shrapnel that wound up scattered throughout the body. It took Patrylak nearly

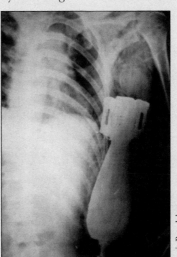

Taken aboard the Sanctuary, *this x-ray shows a mortar shell lodged in a soldier's chest wall.*

Juris Patrylak

a month before he could perform the exam in less than 10 minutes, but unfortunately he had many opportunities to practice.

Patrylak's experiences in Vietnam haunted him for years afterward. "Everyone who was available performed triage when the Jolly Green Giants — the Marine CH-53 helicopters — came in with a load of wounded," Patrylak said. "We'd lay the bodies out on the deck, sorting the live from the dead."

Back in the radiology department, the technologists saw a lot of limb injuries, many of them caused by booby traps. "There were a lot of maimed legs and feet," Patrylak recalled. "The surgeons had to perform many, many amputations."

To save precious time, patients' clothing was removed before they were delivered to the radiology department. One time, however, the patient load was heavy and a soldier arrived fully clothed. As Patrylak began examining the man, he found a hand grenade in the folds of his pants. He quickly called ordnance to dispose of the device. "The radiology department was below the water line, one deck above the bilge," Patrylak said. "If that grenade had gone off, the entire ship would have been in trouble."

The *Sanctuary* sailed to wherever the fighting was heavy. While Patrylak was aboard, the ship moved mainly between Da Nang and the demilitarized zone to the south. Patrylak recalled particularly heavy activity near Hue and China Beach.

The medical crew's primary responsibility was treating U.S. soldiers, but it did provide care to limited numbers of South Vietnamese military and civilians. "A few times we treated Vietcong soldiers because we didn't know who was who," Patrylak said. "As soon as they were stabilized, we got them off the ship." The hardest part, Patrylak said, was treating the South Vietnamese children. "The majority of them had been orphaned by the war. They suffered horribly. It just didn't make any sense."

The statistics reveal the vast toll of the Vietnam War: killed were 58,153 U.S. soldiers, 1.1 million Communist fighters, 223,748 South Vietnamese soldiers and nearly 2 million civilians.

When Patrylak's tour of duty ended in 1971, he returned to Yale-New Haven Hospital as a special procedures technologist and became active in the Connecticut Society of Radiologic Technologists, serving as CSRT president in 1973-74.

In 1974 the CSRT scheduled one of its meetings at a local Veterans Administration Hospital. While walking through the hospital corridors on his way to speak at the meeting, Patrylak was approached by a patient. "You probably don't remember me, but I remember you," the man told Patrylak, extending his hand. "You examined me after I was injured in Vietnam. This is the first chance I've had to say thank you."

—*Ceela McElveny*

requirements. As soon as there were enough two-year schools to satisfy the demand for new trainees, the ASRT and ACR recommended that only graduates of AMA-approved schools be eligible for certification by the Registry. The culmination of nearly 50 years' worth of effort toward establishing suitable educational requirements for technologists came on July 1, 1966, when the Registry began restricting certification to graduates of AMA-approved programs.

The need for formal education was obvious. Of the 2,929 candidates who took the November 1965 Registry exam in x-ray technology, 83.9 percent of those who were graduates of AMA-approved programs passed the exam, while only 57.8 percent of those who were informally trained passed the exam.

Nevertheless, some complained about the new educational requirements. ASRT President Patricia J. O'Reilly, R.T., addressed their concerns in a 1964 editorial in *Radiologic Technology*. She wrote, "The Registry figures will attest to the fact that the formally trained, even under today's still imperfect programs,

edge out the office trainee. Even if this were not a fact, continuance of an apprentice-type training can do nothing but restrict the progress of technology."

The technologists who fought for higher educational standards understood that their profession was fueled by knowledge. Despite their efforts, however, many physicians and hospitals continued to employ undereducated personnel to staff their radiology departments. Society leaders gradually became convinced that to rid the profession of lesser-trained technologists and improve patient care, it would have to reverse its position on licensure.

The licensure issue caused the profession to become embroiled in politics like never before.

Surprisingly, the dawn of the legal age in radiologic technology occurred in a roundabout way. When Sen. Bob Bartlett of Alaska opened Congressional hearings on x-rays in 1967, he was concerned about radiation leakage from color television sets, not the licensure of x-ray technologists. But by the end of his hearings in 1968, he and others in Congress were convinced of the necessity for licensing operators of x-ray equipment.

Prior to Bartlett's hearings, the last time Congress had considered legislation affecting radiation workers was in 1959, when it passed a bill authorizing the Atomic Energy Commission to establish training requirements for personnel who came in contact with certain man-made radioactive materials. But in the mid-1960s it was discovered that vacuum tubes used in circuits of color TV receivers could act as x-ray generators, in some instances emitting in excess of 0.5 mr/hour. This discovery prompted Bartlett to introduce Public Law 90-602, the Radiation Control for Health and Safety Act of 1968. The act would authorize the federal government to establish a radiation control program setting limits on certain types of radiation-emitting equipment, including medical devices. During the hearings, some questioned why the equipment should be monitored when its operators were not. Thus, Bartlett's hearings unintentionally opened debate about whether radiologic technologists should be licensed.

Sen. Bartlett invited the ASRT to testify before Congress on the issue. On May 8, 1968, ASRT board member Leslie Wilson, R.T., appeared before the Senate Commerce Committee to support federal minimum standards for the education of radiologic technologists. Wilson acknowledged that the ASRT had for many years opposed any form of government regulation as a means of establishing educational standards, but explained that federal standards had become necessary to drum out technologists who were patently unqualified by lack of experience or education. According to the U.S. Public Health Service, in 1968 there were more than 100,000 operators of x-ray equipment in the United States, but only about 55,000 were certified by the Registry.

"We believe that federal minimum standards for operators of devices that produce ionizing radiation for medical uses are necessary and desirable (1) to prevent a proliferation of standards throughout the country, (2) to aid the states unable to mount their own programs, and (3) to aid in providing a more consistent and constant protection to the public from unnecessary exposure to ionizing radiation," Wilson said. He also recommended that the federal standards be the two-year curriculum espoused by the ASRT, although states would be free to establish more rigid requirements.

A few days after Wilson's testimony, Bartlett added a section to his bill to provide for the licensing of radiologic technologists. This amendment, however, was deleted during conference committee hearings to resolve differences between the House and Senate versions of the bill. Bartlett's bill, minus the licensure provision, was signed by President Johnson on Oct. 18, 1968.

> *This Society will fight to its death to maintain and protect what we feel is justifiably our basis for the training of competent technologists to meet the needs of the patients we serve...*

When Sen. Bartlett died a year later, the licensure mantle was taken up by a man who would prove to be one of the profession's strongest advocates on Capitol Hill — Sen. Jennings Randolph. With the ASRT's backing, the West Virginia Democrat on June 16, 1970, introduced a bill in the Senate to establish federal minimum standards of education for radiologic technologists. It also called on the federal government to develop and issue to the states criteria for the licensure of radiologic technologists. Following the issuance of these standards, the states would have two years either to adopt them or enact their own,

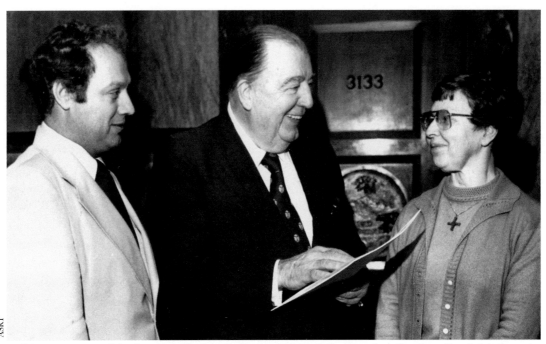

ASRT

1979 *- As sponsor of the Consumer-Patient Radiation Health Safety Act, Sen. Jennings Randolph (center) met with ASRT Executive Director Ward Keller and President Sister Agnes Therese Duffy.*

more stringent, standards.

The ASRT endorsed the bill because it wanted to avoid the possibility of 50 standards for 50 states. New Jersey and California in 1969 joined New York and Puerto Rico in enacting licensure laws for radiologic technologists. The California law particularly worried the Society because it created eight categories of technologists, with training varying from three months to 24 months. Equally alarming was the 1970 amendment of the New York licensure law. To help ease the chronic shortage of x-ray personnel, the New York law was amended to allow schools of radiologic technology to accept students who had neither a high school diploma nor its equivalent. The profession feared that its hard-won educational standards were beginning to unravel. The ASRT asked its affiliate societies to curtail licensure activities in their individual states, if possible, in favor of national licensure.

Sen. Randolph's original bill died in committee. He reintroduced it on Jan. 28, 1971,

and on Jan. 31, 1973. Each time, the bill died when Congress failed to act on it before adjournment. In 1974 the bill was passed by the Senate by a vote of 65 to 18, but failed to make it out of the House Subcommittee on Health. The Senate again approved the legislation on July 1, 1976, as part of the Health Manpower Act, but the licensure provision was deleted during conference committees because the House version of the bill contained no comparable provision. By now, seven states had enacted licensure laws and legislation was pending in several others.

Despite the disappointments on the national front, the ASRT remained optimistic. "This Society will fight to its death to maintain and protect what we feel is justifiably our basis for the training of competent technologists to meet the needs of the patients we serve," President Royce Osborn, R.T., announced in 1970. "We are still firmly convinced that our continuing quest for federal minimum standards through legislative efforts is the right method of approach."

The Essentials

Perhaps the best example of radiologic technologists' growing unity as a profession was the successful conclusion in 1978 of their five-year battle to revise the *Essentials of an Accredited Program for the Radiographer.* Initially adopted in 1944 and revised in 1955 and 1969, the *Essentials* defined the minimum standards for educational programs in radiologic technology.

The 1969 revision required educational programs in the radiologic sciences to be a minimum of 24 months in length — a change that the ASRT, ACR and AMA all supported. That unity disappeared, however, the next time the *Essentials* came up for revision.

The ASRT and JRCERT began rewriting the *Essentials* in 1973. The ACR approved the document in 1976 and passed it along to the AMA. The AMA expressed concern over what it called a lack of sufficient detail concerning curriculum content and returned the draft to the ASRT. In 1977 the ASRT and JRCERT rewrote the draft and again submitted it to the ACR, which approved it in an "emergency action."

The AMA, however, still wasn't satisfied. Its Committee on Allied Health Education and Accreditation made substantial changes to the draft. CAHEA wanted to delete references to the JRCERT as the body responsible for designating maximum student enrollment; delete the JRCERT as the body responsible for recognition of major clinical affiliates of accredited programs; change the definition of program director from an ARRT-registered technologist to a person "qualified in radiography"; and change the definition of the medical director from a "diplomate of the American Board of Radiology" to a "qualified physician."

These changes were not acceptable to the ASRT, but CAHEA responded that they were not open to negotiation.

Thus rebuked, the ASRT called its most powerful weapon — its members — into action. They responded wholeheartedly, deluging CAHEA with more than 2,000 letters and petitions protesting the changes. When CAHEA met in Tampa, Fla., in March 1978, nearly 200 concerned supporters of the ASRT, ARRT, ACR and JRCERT descended upon the meeting. More than 30 of them spoke during the hearing.

"I am convinced that the American Medical Association did not expect either the volume of mail or the number of people who attended the hearing," said 1977-78 ASRT President Richard G. Bauer, R.T. Others agreed. One member wrote the Society, noting, "I have never felt quite as much pride and respect for my professional organization as I did in Tampa. The strategy organized by the ASRT was incredible." Another said, "The feeling of unity and support in that room has never been witnessed in the profession. This may be the beginning of a new era."

Following the hearing, CAHEA representatives agreed to meet with ASRT, ACR and JRCERT leaders to further refine the *Essentials* and reach a compromise on the divisive issues. In doing so, the ASRT prevented the AMA from watering down the minimum qualifications for the positions of program director and medical director.

The AMA finally adopted the *Essentials* on June 16, 1978, and they were implemented in 1980. ASRT Executive Director Ward Keller called the latest revision "a set of standards by which our educational process can evolve to its fullest potential."

—*Ceela McElveny*

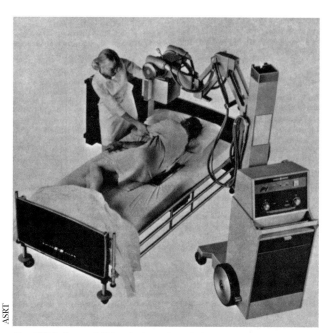

ASRT

In 1970 General Electric introduced the first battery-powered mobile x-ray unit in the United States.

Fortunately, Sen. Randolph had the same opinion. Waiting was nothing new to Randolph; in October 1942 he introduced the first Senate bill to lower the voting age to 18. He had to introduce the legislation 11 more times before it finally was approved by Congress and became law on July 1, 1971.

When the ASRT conducted its Annual Conference in Washington, D.C., in 1977, Randolph was a guest speaker. "It is my earnest hope that we pass this bill, not because I am associated with it, but because of you and those of you who believe in your profession and its healing power," he told ASRT members. The senator received a standing ovation.

While the licensure debate dragged on year after year, another equally contentious issue emerged — the low economic status of radiologic science professionals. Suddenly, the ASRT found itself forced to fight a two-front war.

For many years, money was considered a dirty word by members of the health pro-

fessions. That attitude changed in the late 1960s, when medical workers announced that although they were dedicated to serving humanity, they also expected to be paid a living wage. Until 1966, employees of nonprofit hospitals were not covered under the Fair Labor Standards Act, which enforced the federal minimum wage. A 1967 survey showed that average monthly salaries for staff technologists in diagnostic x-ray were some of the lowest among health professionals — $446 for men and $401 for women. Even worse, the gap between x-ray technologists and other health workers was widening. In 1966 registered nurses averaged $200 more per year than registered technologists; by 1972 the salary difference between the two groups had increased to $1,200 per year.

Frustrated, many medical workers turned to labor unions for help. Unions in hospitals were virtually nonexistent prior to the 1960s. By 1967, however, 8 percent of the nation's 7,172 hospitals had union contracts and by 1970 almost 15 percent of U.S. hospital employees were represented by a union. A sign of the times, the American Nurses Association revoked its long-standing "no-strike" pledge in the mid-1960s and began to use techniques such as mass resignations and "sick-outs" to gain representation in hospitals.

Although the ASRT refused to resort to such drastic measures, it could not ignore the economic plight of its members. The Society's traditional function was to establish and maintain high standards of education. At the 1968 Annual Conference in Los Angeles, however, the Society broadened its philosophy. Members voted to amend the bylaws to state that one of the purposes and functions of the Society would be to improve the welfare and socioeconomic status of radiologic technologists. The ASRT pledged to work on issues of economic concern and actively seek improved salaries, working conditions and fringe benefits.

Despite its new philosophy, the ASRT remained firmly opposed to unionization. "Unions view the R.T. as an untapped financial resource to be added to their list of dues-paying members," read a report in a 1972 issue of the Society newsletter, the *ASRT Scanner.* "The motivations of unions which represent the unskilled labor market are in no way compatible with the interests and goals of professional medical personnel."

The Society recognized the right of hospital employees to organize, but refused to become the collective bargaining agent for radiologic technologists. "To call the ASRT a union is no more true than it is to call the AMA a union," Executive Director Robert Best said in 1971. However, the Society did become embroiled in several bitter employee relations cases. For example, the ASRT supported the 1972 efforts of technologists who filed a complaint with the National Labor Relations Board charging the Ochsner Clinic in New Orleans of unfair labor practices. The clinic refused to meet with technologists to discuss salaries, even though they had formed a bargaining organization known as the Social Economic Organization for Staff Radiologic Technologists. The NLRB found the clinic guilty of unfair labor practices and issued an order requiring the clinic to bargain with the technologists.

The ASRT had to balance its stance against unions with its members' needs. In 1972 it joined the National Economic Council of Associations of Health Professions, a voluntary nonprofit association established to provide organizational assistance to health care workers who wanted to engage in collective bargaining with their employers. The NEC wasn't a collective bargaining agent, but it helped establish chapters that acted as bargaining agents. In retaliation, some hospitals made every effort to discourage membership

THE WHITE HOUSE
July 18, 1969

Dear Mr. Best,

It was most thoughtful of the American Society of Radiologic Technologists to remember me in such a special way at a recent convention meeting. Although I was absent from the city and missed an opportunity to send greetings to the members at the closing session, I am deeply grateful for the expression of friendship represented by the honor extended to me.

With appreciation and best wishes to you and the members of the Society,

Sincerely,
Patricia Nixon

Mr. Robert Best
Executive Director
American Society of Radiologic
Technologists
645 North Michigan Avenue
Chicago, Illinois 60611

ASRT

During the 1969 Annual Conference, ASRT members bestowed honorary membership upon First Lady Patricia Nixon, who worked as an x-ray technologist before her marriage.

in the ASRT.

While wages for radiologic technologists as a group were low, they were even lower for female members of the profession. Despite federal legislation requiring equal pay for equal work, sex discrimination still was common in the business world. A 1971 ASRT survey showed average annual salaries of radiologic technologists were $7,759 for men but only $6,795 for women who performed identical work — a $964 differential. A second survey that year showed that although women dominated the profession in numbers, they held 70 percent of the lower-paying staff technologist positions and only 36 percent of the upper level positions such as chief technologist and assistant chief technologist.

The low salaries impacted the profession in

many ways. Because they were not paid well, many radiologic technologists had self-image problems. They did not view themselves as professionals and did not see a need to join their professional society. As a result, membership in the ASRT stagnated. In 1967-68 the Society represented nearly 30 percent of technologists registered by the ARRT. By 1971-72 that figure dipped to less than 15 percent.

The membership decline put the Society in a precarious financial situation. In 1970, with membership hovering near 8,000, the ASRT launched an aggressive recruitment drive. President Leslie Wilson, R.T., warned that unless membership figures rose, the Society would have to curtail its activities — activities that benefited all radiologic technologists, not just members. The appeal worked and membership figures climbed during the 1970s, reaching 11,000 in early 1973 and 15,000 by the beginning of 1976. The 1975 Annual Conference in San Francisco drew 2,500 attendees, setting a new record.

The Society also launched a massive public relations campaign in 1971, including a series of image-building radio announcements recorded by two popular television actors of the era, Lorne Green of "Bonanza" fame and Jim Nabors of "Gomer Pyle." The goal was to build nationwide public recognition for radiologic technologists and recruit more people to the profession.

Wages, however, remained dismal. "Why are salaries low?" ASRT member Bill Conklin, R.T., asked in a 1972 issue of the *ASRT Scanner*. "Lack of professionalism." Conklin noted that only 15 percent of registered radiologic technologists were members of the ASRT, while 91 percent of physicians belonged to the AMA and 75 percent of eligible radiologists belonged to the ACR. He also laid blame for the low salaries at the feet of a persistent problem: the lack of uniformity in educational programs.

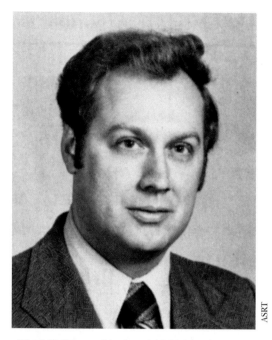

Ward Keller was hired as ASRT director of education in 1974 and took over as executive director of the Society in 1976.

The Society and ACR, still grappling with this old issue, formed the Joint Review Committee on Educational Programs in Radiologic Technology in 1969. The JRCERT was charged with the responsibility of surveying schools of radiologic technology and making recommendations to the accrediting body, the AMA Council on Medical Education. The original JRCERT board was comprised of three radiologic technologists appointed by the ASRT and three radiologists appointed by the ACR.

In 1973 Robert Coyle resigned his position as ASRT director of education to become executive director of the JRCERT. On Jan. 28, 1974, Ward M. Keller, R.T., was hired to replace Coyle as the Society's director of education. Keller, certified by the Registry in 1967, previously was director of education at St. Mary of Nazareth Hospital Center's School of Radiologic Technology in Chicago, Ill. Keller had served on many ASRT committees and was especially interested in radiologic sciences education. He was instrumental in the 1969 creation of the JRCERT and was chairman of the task force that began revising the radiography curriculum in 1971.

Under Keller's direction, the ASRT began discussing a voluntary continuing education program in which technologists could earn CE points by participating in professional meetings, in-service education and self-study programs. Each clock hour of attendance or participation would be worth 1 CE point. The Society's Evidence of Continuing Education (ECE) program formally was instituted before the end of 1974.

With the creation of the ECE program, the Society on April 28, 1975, hired Marilyn Fay, R.T., as its director of continuing education. She had been the director of education at Morristown Memorial Hospital in Morristown, N.J. The Society began developing CE materials that included videotapes, slides, cassettes, textbooks and homestudies. It also sponsored educational institutes — two- or three-day seminars focusing on various topics —throughout the country.

Response to the voluntary continuing education program was strong. In April 1975, 540 people were enrolled in the ECE program. By October 1976 the number had grown to more than 5,000, a testament to technologists' eagerness for continuing education.

Growth at the Registry continued as well. The number of examinees increased every year, forcing the Registry in 1972 to contract Educational Testing Services of Princeton, N.J., for the independent administration and scoring of ARRT examinations. "The Registry is no longer an informal business," said executive director Roland McGowan in announcing the shift. To assist in the construction of its exams, the Registry in 1974 established item writing committees in each category of certification. In 1979 the Registry began cooperating with state licensing agencies to implement state credentialing or licensing exams for radiologic technologists, eventually leading to the ARRT administering its examinations to candidates for state licensure.

Also in 1979 the Registry hired Jerry Reid, Ph.D., as its first director of psychometric services. Reid had earlier that year received his doctorate in educational measurement from Pennsylvania State University. As the 1970s drew to a close, the Registry worked closely with the ASRT and JRCERT to advance the radiologic technologist's status and education.

In 1976 Ward Keller was promoted to executive director of the ASRT. During the next several years, Keller presided over some of the most contentious debates the profession had ever faced, including the very right to call its members professionals.

In 1979 the ASRT petitioned the National Labor Relations Board to change the radiologic technologist's status from "technical" to "professional." Technologists were supported in their efforts by the ACR, which in 1980 adopted a statement recognizing radiologic technologists "as professional members of the health care team." The NLRB, however, would not agree to a general rule change. It said the Society would have to present test cases proving that technologists practiced independently, had specialized knowledge and standards of practice, and restricted entrance into their profession through education, certification and licensure.

The profession again found itself pinning its hopes on licensure, this time as a route to professional status. Sen. Jennings Randolph reintroduced his licensure bill, now titled the Consumer-Patient Radiation Health and Safety Act, in 1978 and 1979. ASRT President Daniel P. Donohue, R.T., was called before the House Subcommittee on Oversight and Investigations on July 24, 1979. He testified, "There are an estimated 130,000 to 170,000 operators of medical x-ray equipment in the United States. Of these, approximately 80,000 have demonstrated their competence through voluntary certification or state licensing examining. The remaining 50,000 to 90,000 have no recognized credential.... Only nine states in the nation have seen fit to regulate or require licensure of individuals who operate this potentially dangerous equipment. In the more than 40 non-regulated states, anyone, and I literally mean anyone, can operate this equipment."

Those who opposed licensure, however, were able to exert more political pressure than those who supported it.

The main source of opposition to national licensure came from the ACR and the AMA. In 1974 James P. Steele, M.D., chairman of the ACR Commission on Radiologic Technology, testified before the Senate Labor and Public Welfare Committee. "As the supervisors of most technologists," Steele said, "radiologists have reason to believe that they, more than another group, can define the skills, qualifications and levels of training required of their helpers." The ACR opposed federal licensure of radiologic technologists for a number of reasons, but primary among them was the ACR's belief that licensure would create hardships for rural hospitals that could not obtain and employ adequately educated technologists. The ACR also opposed the licensure bill because it did not include a provision for "limited permit" technologists with less education.

The ASRT was firm in its opposition to these "limited permitees." As Jean Widger, R.T., stated in a 1978 editorial in *Radiologic Technology*, it was as if the ACR and AMA were saying, "OK, license them, but license some of them only in those examinations that we need to have done in our offices and clinics." By 1978 the California licensure law, for example, had nine limited permit classifica-

tions — chest, gastrointestinal, genitourinary, leg, musculoskeletal, photofluorographic chest, skull, extremities and dental. This created the odd categories of "leg technologists" and "skull technologists" who were licensed to perform only one particular type of x-ray examination. "As long as nonradiologists continue to have x-ray equipment in their offices, the physician will find a justification for the limited permittee," Widger wrote.

The licensure tide finally began to turn in the profession's favor in 1980, when Ward Keller and Daniel Donohue returned to Washington to testify before a Senate subcommittee on health and scientific research. Donohue said, "We remain firm in our opinion that without uniform national standards for qualifications of medical radiation technologists, the public will remain unprotected and at the mercy of untrained personnel." The bill passed unanimously in the Senate. A few months later, Keller returned to Washington with ASRT President Marilyn Holland, R.T., to testify before the House of Representatives. Time ran out before the House voted on the bill, however, and once again it died in committee.

On Feb. 16, 1981, Sen. Randolph reintroduced the licensure bill in the Senate and a month later it was reintroduced in the House. Closer than ever to gaining passage, the ASRT mobilized its membership, launching a massive letter-writing campaign to Congress during the spring of 1981.

As Congressional debate on the legislation came down to the wire that summer, Keller was faced with a difficult decision: either change the mandatory licensure provision to an "advisory" status or risk defeat of the entire bill. "I remember it was my birthday, Aug. 13, when I received a phone call from our legislative rep," Keller said. "He was calling me from the cloak room of the Senate and said we had to make a decision whether to make the bill voluntary or mandatory. They were going to vote that night. It was supposed to be mandatory licensure in all the states, but we knew it wouldn't pass," Keller said. "I said go voluntary. It passed that night."

After 13 years of effort, the Consumer-Patient Radiation Health and Safety Act of 1981, Subtitle 1 of Public Law 97-35, was passed by both houses of Congress and signed by President Ronald Reagan on Aug. 13, 1981. The act required the Secretary of Health and Human Services to develop federal standards for the certification of radiologic technologists and the accreditation of educational programs in radiologic technology. It also required the federal government to provide the states with a model statute for licensure. Compliance by states was voluntary, and the act did not impose penalties for states that ignored the standards.

By 1995, 33 states had enacted licensure laws, many in accordance with the model statute provided by the federal government.

In recognition of his efforts, Sen. Jennings Randolph was made an honorary member of the ASRT at the 1982 Annual Conference.

The passage of the Radiation Health and Safety Act was a watershed event in the profession's history, officially establishing the importance of education and certification to the radiologic sciences. More importantly, this hard-won victory proved that with a solid foundation of knowledge, a commitment to goals and a belief in their capabilities, radiologic technologists could accomplish anything.

Bringing Hope to the World

Radiologic technologists are known for a willingness to share not only their medical skills, but also their medical knowledge. In the 1960s and '70s, dozens of them took advantage of a unique opportunity to do both.

It had long been the dream of Washington, D.C., heart specialist William B. Walsh, M.D., to bring modern U.S. health care techniques to the citizens of developing nations. In 1958 Walsh met with President Dwight D. Eisenhower to discuss ideas for what he called "Project Hope," an acronym for "Health Opportunities for People Everywhere." Two years later, Walsh's project was launched — literally. The *S.S. Hope*, the world's first peacetime hospital ship and medical training center, left Baltimore in 1960 for her first medical mission in Indonesia.

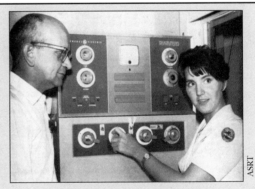

Department chief Malcolm Metcalf, R.T., and technologist Caroline Strong Steele, R.T., worked on the S.S. Hope *during its 1964 mission to Ecuador.*

During the next two decades, the *Hope* and its team of medical experts traveled to countries throughout the world with a double mission: treatment and training. Its staff provided free medical care for the underprivileged while sharing U.S. medical knowledge with local health care providers.

The *S.S. Hope's* impact on world health conditions was immeasurable. By 1972 the seafaring medical clinic had visited Indonesia, South Vietnam, Peru, Ecuador, Guinea,

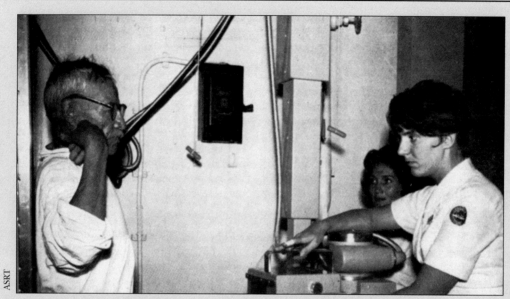

ASRT

Steele, far right, teaches her Ecuadoran counterpart while performing an x-ray examination of a Ecuadorian patient.

West Africa, Nicaragua, Columbia, Ceylon, Tunisia and the Caribbean Islands. Its medical staff had treated more than 120,000 people, performed more than 10,000 surgeries and trained 4,000 local physicians, surgeons, dentists, nurses and technologists.

Many U.S. radiologic technologists served aboard the *Hope*, either as one of its 120 permanent staff or as a member of the rotating team of health specialists who signed up for two- or three-month tours of duty.

The ship's radiology department had all the latest technology. It was comprised of a diagnostic x-ray room, a special procedures room, a viewing room and a darkroom that featured an automatic film processor. All the radiology equipment had been donated by U.S. manufacturers, including General Electric and Kodak. Veronica Durichek, R.T., who served aboard the floating hospital during its mission to Tunisia in 1970 and to the Caribbean and Latin America in 1971, called the department's equipment "better than anything I ever had to work with in the states."

The ship was welcomed with enthusiasm at its various ports of call. Caroline Strong Steele, R.T., who served on the *Hope* during its 1964 mission to Latin America, later recalled that "every person in Ecuador wanted to be a patient on the *Hope*." Many people from the country's small villages had never before been examined by a doctor, Steele explained. While docked in Ecuador, the Hope vaccinated 143,000 people against polio and 133,000 children against diphtheria. In addition, every patient received a chest radiograph to screen for tuberculosis.

Although the *Hope* provided extensive free medical attention to people of developing countries, its main purpose was teaching. As part of the *Hope's* mission to upgrade the skills of local medical professionals, every North American physician, nurse and technologist aboard the ship was expected to train a local counterpart. Durichek taught diagnostic and radioisotope procedures during her mission to Tunisia, while Steele taught diagnostic procedures to her counterpart in Ecuador. There were no schools for nursing, radiologic technology or laboratory technology in Ecuador at the time. People holding these positions in Ecuadorian hospitals were expected to learn their skills on the job. Still, Steele said her counterpart "misunderstood her mission and thought she was to teach us!"

After the *Hope* ended its medical mission in a country, a small North American staff of nurses, a laboratory technologist and an x-ray technologist stayed behind to work in the local hospital and set up a permanent teaching program. This shore staff would remain in the country until the local hospital could operate without the help of the North Americans.

Malcolm Metcalf, R.T., who served for five years as the *Hope's* chief radiologic technologist, said teaching was stressed because it allowed the *Hope* to have a more enduring effect on local health conditions than would attempts at widespread treatment.

Metcalf, who traveled to four continents during his tenure on the Hope, learned how to say "Take a deep breath and hold it" in French, Spanish, Quechua, Jibaro, Malinke, Soussou and Foulani. When he later wrote about his experiences, Metcalf called his work on the ship "the most enjoyable and fulfilling I've ever encountered."

By the time the *S.S. Hope* was retired from duty in 1977, its crew had brought immunization, diagnosis and treatment to more than 3 million people around the globe. Project Hope continued into the 1980s as a land-based operation, establishing medical training centers throughout the world.

For the radiologic technologists who were part of Project Hope, work meant more than just a paycheck. They helped bring medical knowledge and treatment to people who needed it the most — all as part of a project as promising as the name given it.

—*Ceela McElveny*

Chapter Ten

The Healing Rays

The medical profession advanced rapidly following Roentgen's discovery of the x-ray. Virtually every aspect of medicine came to rely on radiology in some way, and for the first time surgical planning could be based on knowledge gained before an operation. But the x-ray not only revolutionized diagnostic medicine, it transformed therapeutic medicine as well. Only months after its discovery, the x-ray was being used to heal injuries and cure disease.

As its technology grew in sophistication, radiation therapy evolved into a separate specialty in its own right. Today it is the cornerstone of cancer management programs throughout the world. Nearly 60 percent of U.S. cancer patients are treated with some form of radiation therapy to relieve pain and prolong life. Radiation therapists — the health professionals who deliver this life-saving treatment — form the front lines in the battle against cancer.

Because Roentgen's experiments with x-rays were widely duplicated and put to immediate medical use in both Europe and America, the first therapeutic use of radiation is difficult to pinpoint. Chicago medical student and lamp manufacturer Emil H. Grubbé claimed he employed x-rays to treat a carcino-ma of the breast on Jan. 29, 1896 — just weeks after the public announcement of Roentgen's discovery. During the month of January 1896, Grubbé tested dozens of Crookes tubes for x-ray production, exposing his left hand to radiation for between 150 and 200 hours. He developed severe dermatitis and sought treatment at Hahnemann Medical College, where a physician named J.E. Gilman questioned Grubbé about the cause of the damage.

Learning that Grubbé had been experimenting with x-rays, Gilman told his patient, prophetically, that "any physical agent capable of doing so much damage to normal or healthy cells and tissues might offer possibilities, if used as a therapeutic measure, in the treatment of pathological conditions."

This comment intrigued Grubbé, who on Jan. 29 had an opportunity to investigate the theory. When a patient with a carcinoma of the breast was referred to his office, Grubbé placed an x-ray tube close to the lesion and exposed it to radiation for almost an hour. "For the first time in history, x-rays had been used for treatment, not diagnostic purposes," Grubbé wrote of his accomplishment in 1933. "That was the beginning of the treatment of diseases with x-rays; that was the origin of x-ray therapy."

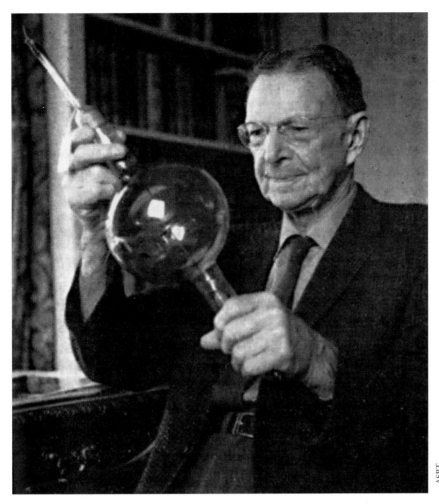

ASRT

The 1913 development of the Coolidge hot cathode tube made higher voltage x-ray treatment possible. William Coolidge posed with his invention in 1967, at the age of 94.

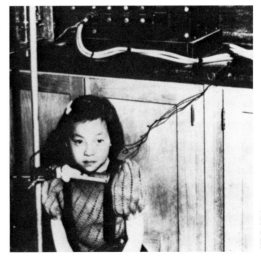

Following World War II, reactor-produced radioisotopes became widely available. This young patient's thyroid function is being measured with Iodine 131 and a Geiger counter.

HP Publishers

Grubbé performed a total of 18 x-ray treatments on his patient. Unfortunately, the therapy showed no beneficial effects and the patient died within a month.

Although there is some dispute over the accuracy of Grubbé's claim to be the father of radiation therapy, it is known that x-rays were being used for therapeutic purposes within months after their discovery. In July and August 1896 a French physician named V. Despeignes experimented with x-rays to treat a gastric carcinoma. Later that fall Dr. J. William White, a professor of clinical surgery at the University of Pennsylvania, began investigating x-rays as a possible cure for cancer.

These early experiments showed promise, but real proof of the x-ray's healing power came unexpectedly. By 1897 physicians knew that lengthy exposures to radiation caused hair to fall out. They began using x-rays to treat excessive hair growth, especially on women's faces. In 1900 Dr. William Allen Pusey, a dermatology professor in Chicago, discovered that x-rays not only eliminated one patient's excess facial hair, it also cured her acne.

Immediately after this discovery, physicians rushed to use the x-ray as a treatment for skin diseases such as skin tuberculosis (lupus vulgaris) and skin cancer. Obtaining favorable results, they soon began applying x-rays to cancers of the breast, uterus, rectum, intestine, neck and head. By 1902 Heber Robarts, founder of the American Roentgen Ray Society, announced there were "about 100 named diseases that yield favorably to x-ray treatment." The era of radiation therapy had

> **❛**
> *Marie Curie's 1898 discovery of radium and its radioactive properties gave rise to "curie therapy," the precursor of modern brachytherapy. As early as 1903, radium-filled glass "seeds" or needles were placed on or inside patients' bodies to cure disease.*
> **❜**

begun in earnest.

Initially, the same x-ray tubes were used for diagnosis and therapy. The generators and Crookes tubes available before 1910 were capable of producing x-rays of relatively low energy, ranging only between 50 kilovolts and 100 kilovolts. These low voltages produced an x-ray beam of poor penetrating power, limiting the applicability of x-rays for the treatment of cancer and other diseases. As a result, physicians also began using radiation of a different form — encapsulated radium — to treat cancer.

Marie Curie's 1898 discovery of radium and its radioactive properties gave rise to "curie therapy," the precursor of modern brachytherapy. As early as 1903, radium-filled glass "seeds" or needles were placed on or inside patients' bodies to cure disease. This type of therapy, although often effective, was not without its difficulties. The primary concern was the scarcity of radium itself. Up to 500 tons of uranium or carnotite ore and 2,000 tons of sandstone and rock had to be sifted to mine 1 gram of radium. As a result, radium was extremely limited in supply and expensive; it cost $120,000 per gram in 1903. Even after large amounts of uranium ore were discovered in the Belgian Congo in 1922, radium prices remained above $70,000 per gram.

In addition, radium therapy worked best for skin cancers and easily reached internal tumors. Cancers that lay deep within the body still were inaccessible except through surgery. Until higher energy beams became available, however, interstitial and intracavitary radium therapy was more common than superficial external beam therapy.

That situation changed with the 1913 introduction of the Coolidge hot cathode tube. Invented by William Coolidge, a researcher at General Electric, the Coolidge tube ushered in a new era in diagnostic and therapeutic radiology. Its predecessor, the unpredictable Crookes tube, was gas-filled. Coolidge's invention, by contrast, was a near-perfect vacuum tube that could tolerate higher voltages and, therefore, generate more penetrating x-rays. The first Coolidge tubes could produce 100,000-volt x-rays; they later were improved to generate 200,000-volt x-rays. The Coolidge tube quickly became standard equipment for "deep" or orthovoltage radiation therapy, allowing physicians to deliver powerful — and sometimes curative — doses of radiation directly to a tumor site. The first American deep therapy x-ray unit was made by General Electric for Dr. James T. Case of Battle Creek, Mich., in 1921.

William Coolidge also helped pave the way for supervoltage x-ray machines. By the early 1930s, generators were capable of producing energies of 500,000 volts and higher. To accommodate such powerful voltages, which would destroy a typical x-ray tube, Coolidge invented "cascading" tubes. Under the cascade principle, a portion of the total energy was applied to a series of sections comprising the tube.

One of the first researchers to direct supervoltage x-rays into the human body was Dr. Albert Soiland of Los Angeles. In 1930 Soiland conducted clinical tests on a patient with an adenocarcinoma of the rectum, using a beam of 600,000 volts. The patient's tumor decreased in size.

The first supervoltage unit placed into everyday operation was installed in 1937 at St. Bartholomew's Hospital in London. Requiring a tube 30 feet long, the unit's installation was a major technological achievement. It was capable of 1 million volts of energy and continued to be used into the 1950s.

Occurring almost simultaneously was the development of the betatron and cyclotron, powerful new particle accelerators able to generate up to 20 million volts of energy.

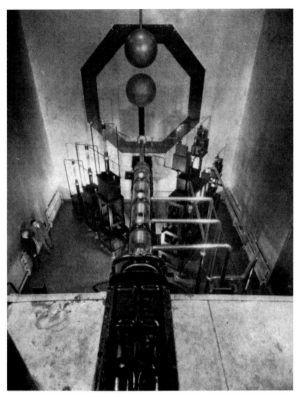

General Electric

William Coolidge pioneered the "cascade" principle used in multisection tubes, such as this 800 kVp therapy unit installed by General Electric at Mercy Hospital in 1933.

These supervoltage units produced x-rays capable of delivering a high radiation dose to tissues deep within the body. The betatron and cyclotron also permitted the use of multiple fields — the crossfire technique — resulting in even higher dosages. However, because effective beam limitation and shielding techniques had not been devised, many radiation therapy patients suffered from overexposure to healthy tissue.

The betatron, a circular electron accelerator, was developed in the early 1940s by Dr. Donald Kerst of the University of Illinois. The betatron generated energy by using an electromagnet to spin electrons through a circular glass tube until they almost reached the speed of light. It was developed commercially by the Siemens Manufacturing Company of Germany and the Shimadzu Manufacturing

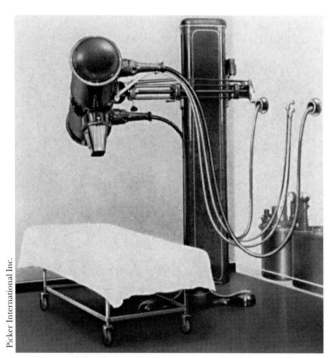

The first all-flexible, shock-proof therapy unit developed by Picker Corporation was installed at the University of Iowa in 1933. It used a Coolidge tube and operated at a maximum of 200 kVp.

Company of Japan, among others.

The cyclotron, based on a similar principle, accelerated protons rather than electrons and generated neutron rays instead of x-rays. It was designed in the early 1930s by Dr. Ernest Lawrence, a physicist at the University of California at Berkeley. To determine whether neutron rays could be used to treat cancer, the first medical cyclotron was tested in 1939 on the Berkeley campus. Early results showed that neutron therapy caused some types of tumors to shrink or disappear. This type of therapy was discontinued within a few years, however, when scientists discovered that neutron rays had severe late effects — much more damaging than x-rays — on healthy tissue surrounding the treated area.

While U.S. researchers were investigating methods of generating ever-higher voltages, a French discovery again changed the direction of radiation therapy. In 1933 Frédéric Joliot

and his future wife Irene Curie, the daughter of Marie and Pierre Curie, discovered artificial radioactivity. While bombarding certain elements with alpha particles from a radioactive source, Joliot and Curie discovered aluminum, boron and magnesium continued to emit positrons even after the radioactive source had been removed. They labeled these altered elements "radioactive isotopes." Within a year of this discovery, researchers found an additional 100 radioactive isotopes. The first therapeutic use of an artificial radioisotope occurred in early 1936 when sodium 24 was administered intravenously to a leukemia patient.

The discovery of artificial radioactivity also created a new use for Lawrence's cyclotron. With its high energy beam, the cyclotron could manufacture radioisotopes in great quantities, thus reducing dependence on naturally-occurring radioactive sources such as radium.

The profession's next major technological advance not only impacted radiation therapy, but also altered world history.

Nuclear fission — the splitting of atoms — was discovered in 1938 in Nazi Germany and later replicated in the United States by a team of scientists from Princeton, Columbia and the University of Chicago. Led by physicist Enrico Fermi, the team succeeded in initiat-

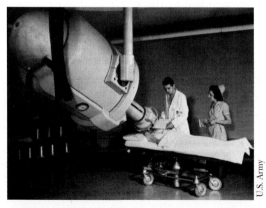

A typical million-volt x-ray therapy unit used early in World War II.

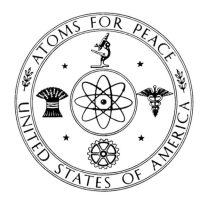 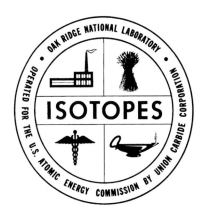

In the 1950s, the nuclear reactor at Oak Ridge National Laboratory was put to use producing medical radioisotopes – part of the Atomic Energy Commission's "Atoms for Peace" program.

ing the first sustained nuclear chain reaction and built the world's first nuclear reactor, leading to the U.S. development and detonation of the atomic bomb. During World War II, nuclear power was harnessed as a destructive force. In the 1950s, however, nuclear reactors were employed for a more peaceful purpose — producing radioisotopes for medical use.

The wave of radioisotope technology took the radiology profession by storm, with the ASXT in 1955 commissioning a series of articles for its journal discussing "where we as technicians will fit into the technical aspects of the radioisotope programs now developing across the country." The ASXT and ARXT wanted to ensure that isotope technology remained within the realm of the radiologic sciences.

The Atomic Energy Commission was created in 1947 and charged by the U.S. government with the responsibility for controlling the production and distribution of radioactive isotopes. Oak Ridge National Laboratory in Tennessee became the world's largest supplier of radionuclides and by 1955 more than 1,200 medical institutions were licensed by the AEC to use reactor-produced isotopes for brachytherapy and tracer studies. Isotopes produced by nuclear reactors were available in larger quantities and at a lower cost than

those produced by cyclotrons.

Radioisotopes also were used as sources of gamma-ray beams for radiation therapy. Gamma rays are emitted when a harmless, stable molecule such as cobalt 59 is converted into an unstable, radioactive molecule such as cobalt 60. Gamma rays are identical to x-rays except in their origin. Cobalt 60 emits gamma rays at 1,170,000 electron volts and 1,350,000 electron volts, providing a source of ionizing radiation that possesses some skin sparing capabilities. The size of the source, however, results in more penumbra than some other treatment methods.

In 1949 Leonard George Grimmett, chief physicist at the M.D. Anderson Hospital and Tumor Institute in Houston, designed a container for the use of cobalt 60 as a radium substitute in teletherapy. The first cobalt 60 unit based on his design was installed in early 1951 at the Saskatoon Cancer Clinic in Canada. That spring, the Oak Ridge Institute for Nuclear Studies began building a 1,000 curie cobalt 60 irradiator for Grimmett. Unfortunately, Grimmett did not witness its 1953 installation at M.D. Anderson; he died of coronary thrombosis in May 1951.

Cobalt 60 and cesium 137 were the most popular sources of supervoltage radiation beams for cancer therapy during the 1950s and '60s. Of the 704 supervoltage units avail-

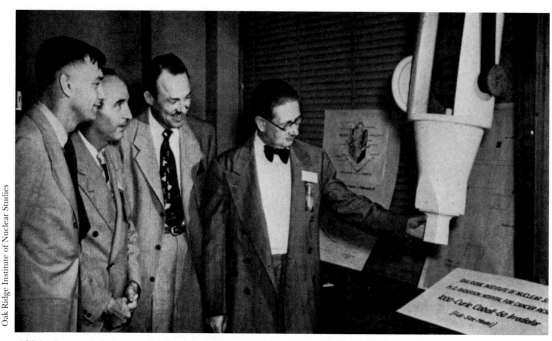

Oak Ridge Institute of Nuclear Studies

1951 - Leonard Grimmett (far right) examines the mock-up of the cobalt 60 unit being built for his radiation therapy program at M.D. Anderson Hospital and Tumor Institute. The unit, one of the first cobalt 60 machines in the United States, was installed in 1953. Grimmett died a few days after this photo was taken.

able in 1968 in the United States and Canada, 623 were cobalt 60 units, 37 were cesium 137 units and the remainder were linear accelerators, betatrons, Van de Graaf units and resonant transformers. Within a few years, however, cobalt units fell out of favor in radiation therapy because of continual improvements in linear accelerators. By the late 1980s, in fact, the medical linear accelerator had eclipsed all other treatment units to become the standard radiation therapy delivery system.

The linear accelerator, or "linac," was invented by William Hansen at Stanford University in the mid-1940s. It was based on research conducted by Russell and Sigurd Varian, the brothers who later founded Varian Associates of Palo Alto, Calif. During World War II, the Varian brothers worked with scientists in the United States and England to design a high-powered microwave tube capable of generating radar signals. Their creation, called a klystron tube, later

became a major component of the linear accelerator. The linac uses microwave energy to accelerate electrons to 186,000 miles per second, nearly the speed of light. As they reach maximum speed, the electrons collide with a metal target and release x-rays.

The linac was first used medically in 1954. It could deliver 10 million volts of energy, but its tube measured more than 6 feet long, making the machine unwieldy to operate. In the mid-1960s the linac tube was downsized by scientists working at Varian Associates so it could be rotated 360° around a reclining patient. The linac's beam penetration was greater than that of earlier orthovoltage systems, making it easier to deliver tumoricidal doses to cancers deep within the body. Its beam also had sharply defined edges so smaller lesions could be treated. The higher radiation dosages made possible by these technological advances made accurate treatment planning and delivery more important than ever.

No longer hampered by inadequate

machinery, the discipline of radiation therapy blossomed in the United States during the '60s and began to establish a distinct identity.

For years, x-ray technologists were responsible for providing diagnostic as well as therapeutic radiology services. The majority of technologists working in radiation therapy had no credentials or formal education and the profession had no distinct recognition or status. Radiation therapy was considered a subspecialty of the diagnostic technologist's duties. In fact, it usually was not a full-time job for most technologists, just an additional responsibility.

In the 1960s, however, physicians began to specialize in radiation therapy and call themselves "radiation therapists" or "radiotherapists" to distinguish themselves from their diagnostic colleagues. Correspondingly, the technologists who actually delivered the treatments began calling themselves "radiation therapy technologists." A new radiologic specialty was emerging. "No longer can a general staff technologist perform efficiently all functions in diagnostic roentgenology, radiation therapy and nuclear medicine," read a report in the ASRT journal in the early 1970s. "Each technologist must 'specialize' as the fields themselves have become specialized."

In 1967 the American Medical Association officially recognized radiation therapy as a distinct discipline from diagnostic imaging. Even into the early 1970s, however, radiation therapy still was considered by some to be an offshoot of diagnostic imaging. In a 1970 lecture before the American Radium Society, Franz Buschke, M.D., said, "Radiation therapy as a specialty has been accepted very reluctantly and is still far from being generally accepted throughout the country. Most of the radiation therapy was, and much still is, performed as an annex to x-ray diagnosis."

In attempting to establish a separate identity from their diagnostic colleagues, technol-

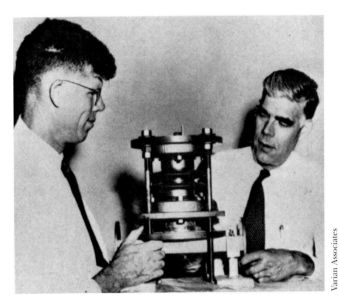

Varian Associates

1939 - The Varian brothers, Russell (left) and Sigurd, inspect a klystron tube. Varian Associates began developing medical linear accelerators in the 1950s, based on the same basic technology as the klystron.

ogists' efforts paralleled physicians'. The Registry created a certification exam for radiation therapy technologists in 1964, 42 years after the first exam in radiography and one year after the first exam in "isotope technology" (nuclear medicine). The first radiation therapy technologists faced a dilemma similar to the first x-ray technologists: little formal education. Still, 108 people sat for the initial Registry examination in radiation therapy, and 88 passed. According to ARRT records, the first person to become credentialed in radiation therapy was Norbert Black, R.T.(R)(T), a therapy technologist at the University of Alabama Hospital in Birmingham. Black credits "alphabetical order" for earning his place in history as the first credentialed radiation therapist. "I was from the state of Alabama and had a last name that began with B," he explained.

The significance of including isotope technologists and radiation therapy technologists under the Registry umbrella was not lost upon the profession. In 1963 ASRT President Patricia O'Reilly, R.T., wrote, "The Registry, with our help and blessing, will certify isotope technologists, and I have heard some question the advisability of such a move. Out of our field? Never. Certification for therapy technologists is but a year away, and not one moment too soon." O'Reilly warned that unless the Registry and ASRT embraced the two newest branches of radiology, splinter groups would emerge and divide the profession.

The first radiation therapy technology curriculum was published in 1964, on the eve of the Registry's implementation of the certification exam. The ASRT Education Committee, which spent two years developing the curriculum, recommended a 12-month course in radiation therapy for technologists already certified in radiography. The curriculum was approved by the American College of Radiology in February 1965. It called for a total of 257 lecture hours, including 60 hours of physics, 25 hours of radium therapy, 70 hours of treatment planning, 12 hours of radiobiology and 15 hours of radiation protection and shielding.

Eileen McCullough, B.H.S., R.T.(R)(T), FASRT, served on the ASRT committee that wrote the curriculum. McCullough was a 1949 graduate of Philadelphia Hospital's School of Radiologic Technology. In 1952 she went to work at the American Oncological Hospital in Philadelphia as a supervoltage therapy technologist and in 1956 she was named chief radiation therapy technologist.

To introduce the radiation therapy technology curriculum, McCullough published an article in the September 1965 issue of *Radiologic Technology*. "In recent years much attention has been focused on the training of the radiologist in therapeutic techniques," she wrote. "Unfortunately, in the United States the training of technologists has not kept

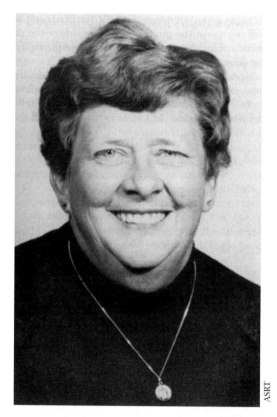

Eileen McCullough was the first recipient of the Varian Award for Achievement in Radiation Therapy Technology.

pace. Now, the need for well-trained assistants to therapeutic radiologists has become acute. It is distressing to learn that many of our leading radiologists are importing technologists and dosimetrists from England and Australia to secure the professional assistance they feel is needed."

Other countries had been quicker than the United States to establish formal educational programs for radiation therapy technologists, and U.S. hospitals establishing therapy departments were not shy in attempting to lure qualified foreign technologists to help develop their fledgling programs. At the time, on-the-job training was the only educational avenue available for most U.S. radiation therapy technologists. By the early 1960s, however, McCullough and a handful of other dedicated technologists were pushing for formalized educational programs.

Many of the first radiation therapy educators in the United States were imports from the United Kingdom. These pioneers included Joyce Lawson, F.S.R., R.T.(T), a 1943 graduate of the School of Radiology Technology in Glasgow, Scotland. Lawson emigrated from Scotland to Canada in 1950 to take a position as a radiation therapy technologist at the London Clinic in Ontario, where she operated one of the first cobalt 60 units in the western hemisphere. In the mid-1950s she was lured to Stanford University in California, where in 1963 she established the first radiation therapy program on the West Coast. Partially funded by the National Cancer Institute, the program followed a two-year curriculum based on Lawson's own training in Glasgow.

Another Scottish import was Margaret Robertson, F.S.R., educated in radiation therapy technology at Glasgow University and the Liverpool Radium Institute. In the mid-1960s Robertson created a two-year radiation therapy curriculum at Mount Sinai School of Medicine in New York, N.Y., and was made responsible for establishing radiation therapy educational criteria for the state.

A third radiation therapy educator emigrating from the United Kingdom was Harold Silverman, R.T.(T). Silverman was educated at Leeds College of Technology in Leeds, England, where he majored in pharmacy. He served as a radiographer in the British Army during World War II, and following the war became certified in radiation therapy by the British Society of Radiographers. In 1964 Silverman brought his British therapy training to the Yale-New Haven Hospital in Connecticut.

Eileen McCullough, the lone American among this group of education pioneers, in 1965 established the Philadelphia School of Radiotherapeutic Technology, sponsored by a consortium of six Philadelphia hospitals.

Through the efforts of educators such as Lawson, Robertson, Silverman and McCullough, the ASRT and ARRT began to make significant inroads toward achieving accreditation of radiation therapy technology programs by the AMA Council on Medical Education. *The Essentials of an Accredited Educational Program for the Radiation Therapy Technologist* were adopted by the AMA in 1968, and in 1969 McCullough's Philadelphia program was the first to earn accreditation. By 1972 the Registry had credentialed more than 600 radiation therapy technologists, and on July 1, 1974, it began restricting the therapy examination to graduates of accredited programs. By July 1, 1975, 1,080 technologists were registered in radiation therapy.

The profession, meanwhile, struggled to standardize its educational programs. At the end of 1975, 61 educational programs had been accredited in radiation therapy technology — 42 offering a one-year curriculum, nine offering a two-year curriculum, and 10 offering a two-year associate degree. The philosophical differences represented by these diverse educational programs resulted in a lack of cohesiveness for radiation therapy technologists.

McCullough's views on how to standardize technologist education differed greatly from Robertson's, particularly on the issue of whether radiation therapy training programs should be one or two years in length. Robertson favored a two-year program, based on her experience in her native Scotland. McCullough preferred a one-year post-radiography program, and funding to test a 12-month curriculum at her Philadelphia school was provided by the U.S. Department of Health, Education and Welfare. Also supporting the 12-month program was the first set of *Essentials*, written by McCullough and Jules Rominger, M.D., and used to evaluate educa-

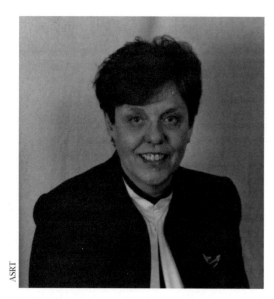

ASRT

Phyllis Thompson was the first radiation therapy technologist on the ASRT Board of Directors. She was elevated to ASRT Fellow in 1985 and received the Varian Award in 1986.

tional programs for accreditation.

The curriculum of the 12-month program was designed for students who previously had completed a two-year educational program in x-ray technology or who already were certified by the Registry in radiography or nuclear medicine. Because the profession faced a severe personnel shortage during the 1970s, however, many educators and hospital administrators pushed for a 24-month educational program that would open radiation therapy technology to high school graduates with no previous education in the radiologic sciences.

To accommodate schools that wanted to implement a longer curriculum, in 1973 a second set of *Essentials* was developed for 24-month programs. When the *Essentials* were revised again in 1976, they continued to state that "educational programs of 24 months and 12 months may be developed."

Still, the debate continued over program length. In 1979 JRCERT chairman Jules Rominger and staff consultant Diana Browning, M.B.A., R.T.(T), wrote, "The 12-month program in radiation therapy technology has led to an erroneous concept in the minds of some that radiation therapy is continuing education for radiographers, and this has placed it in a category with special procedures, computed tomography and ultrasound. Radiation therapy technology is a specialty and should be considered parallel to radiography and nuclear medicine technology."

Rominger and Browning argued that 24-month educational programs, "because they provide technologists with maximum educational exposure in radiation therapy in a shorter overall time," were necessary to help eliminate the chronic personnel shortage and should become the standard for the profession. They encouraged 12-month programs to consider lengthening their curricula.

Others, however, said the personnel shortage was a poor argument in favor of 24-month programs. "In 1977, a 12-month program student capacity of 321 rendered 159 (49.5 percent) applications for ARRT examination," Arlene Caughron, R.T.(R), wrote in the November 1979 issue of *Radiologic Technology*. "For the same period, however, a 24-month program student capacity of 351 students rendered only 103 (29.3 percent) applications to the ARRT."

The issue of program length never was resolved fully, and 12- and 24-month programs existed side-by-side through the 1981, 1988 and 1994 revisions of the *Essentials*. In addition, many schools expanded to include associate and baccalaureate degree programs.

McCullough's Philadelphia program, coming under the sponsorship of Gwynedd-Mercy College in 1975, developed one of the first two-year associate degree programs for radiation therapy technologists. By the mid-1980s the Gwynedd-Mercy program was the largest in the country, educating more than 15 percent of all U.S. radiation therapy technologists. In recognition of McCullough's many achievements, in 1984 she became the first recipient of the Varian Award for Achievement in Radiation Therapy Technology. Following her death in 1989, the award was retitled to include McCullough's name.

For Phyllis Thompson, R.T.(R)(T), FASRT, the 1970s were the period of greatest growth for the profession. Describing that tumultuous decade during her 1986 Varian Award lecture, Thompson said, "Equipment and physics became more complex and so too did treatment planning and delivery. Technologists required more education to cope with the increased responsibility and complex treatment techniques. Our clinical skills quickly surpassed those of the physicians and we became solely responsible for the treatment of patients, causing an increased stratification of duties."

Also during the 1970s, the ASRT began offering educational institutes — two- or three-day seminars — dedicated solely to radiation therapy. Those seminars were phased out in 1977 when radiation therapy technologists began conducting annual conjoint meetings with the physicians' organization, the American Society of Therapeutic Radiologists. The physicians' society later changed its name to the American Society for Therapeutic Radiology and Oncology (ASTRO).

The decade ended with radiation therapy technologists gaining new recognition and status in the radiologic science community. In 1979 Mattie Tabron, Ed.D., R.T.(T), FASRT, became the first radiation therapy technologist to serve on the Registry Board of Trustees. Also that year Phyllis Thompson was elected ASRT vice president, making her the first radiation therapy technologist on the ASRT Board of Directors, and Carole Sullivan, Ph.D., R.T.(R)(T), FASRT, became the first therapy technologist elevated to ASRT Fellow.

In 1980 the first Radiation Therapy Curriculum Guide was published. The list of

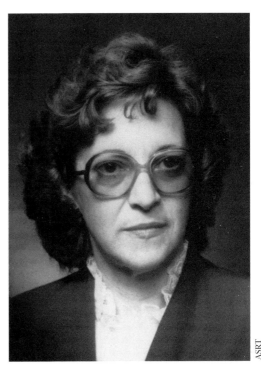

In 1988, Beverly Buck became the first radiation therapist to serve as president of the ASRT.

ASRT task force members who wrote the curriculum guide reads like a "who's who" of radiation therapists; it included Diane Chadwell, R.T.(T); Sheryl Janiec, R.T.(T); Joyce Lawson; Charles Marschke, R.T.(T); and Elizabeth Snyder, R.T.(T). Additional contributions were made by Randall Brown, R.T.(T); Elona McLees, R.T.(T); Diana Browning and Phyllis Thompson.

The first radiation therapy technologist to serve as ASRT president was Beverly A. Buck, R.T.(R)(T), who led the Society during 1988-89. The following year the ASRT hired its first director of radiation therapy education, Lynda Reynolds, B.S., R.T.(R)(T)(N), CNMT. At the time, radiation therapists made up about 13 percent of the ASRT's 16,500 membership.

In the late 1980s physicians who specialized in cancer treatment began calling themselves "radiation oncologists" instead of "radiation therapists." The technologists assumed the title of "radiation therapist,"

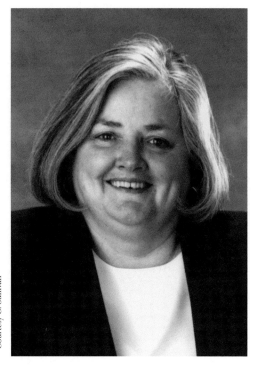

Courtesy C. Sullivan

Carole Sullivan served as chairman of the ASRT Task Force on Educational Standards for Radiation Therapists during 1991-92.

believing it better reflected their duties and responsibilities. Because they were providing primary patient care in addition to delivering treatment, the term "technologist" no longer seemed appropriate. In 1988 the ASRT House of Delegates adopted a resolution to change the job title from "radiation therapy technologist" to "radiation therapist." The ACR, however, was concerned this title change would create confusion among the public and asked the ASRT to reconsider the change or delay its implementation. Therapists discussed and rejected the ACR's request during the 1988 ASRT Radiation Therapy Conference. According to Beverly Buck, "The consensus was that the House of Delegates adopted the title change based on the wishes of the radiation therapy technology community and no further discussion (was) necessary."

The Registry and JRCERT endorsed the therapists' position and reformatted their documents to comply with the change in terminology. In 1994 the ASRT House of Delegates further reinforced the title change, approving a resolution that officially adopts "radiation therapy" as the name of the discipline. Professional status for the discipline's practitioners, however, remained elusive.

The U.S. Department of Labor classified all radiologic technologists, including radiation therapists, as technical workers. Because the Department of Labor's definition of a "professional" included "learning customarily acquired by a prolonged course of specialized intellectual instruction and study," radiation therapists pinned their hopes on the baccalaureate degree as a possible method of achieving professional status. Studies showed that more therapists were obtaining bachelor's degrees; a 1986 survey by the Registry showed that 43 percent of registered radiation therapists held a high school diploma, 36 percent received an associate's degree, 15 percent earned a baccalaureate degree and 2 percent held a master's degree. The remaining 4 percent held doctoral degrees or did not answer the question. But was the profession ready for a mandatory baccalaureate?

That question was first raised publicly during an open forum at the 1990 ASRT Radiation Therapy Conference, held in conjunction with the annual ASTRO meeting. At the 1991 ASRT Annual Conference in Albuquerque, N.M., radiation therapy delegates again met to discuss recognition of radiation therapists as professionals by governmental agencies and external organizations. Following debate of the issue, they wrote a resolution directing the ASRT to initiate a national discussion on elevating entry-level educational standards for therapists. The resolution, adopted by the House of Delegates, asked the ASRT to seek the "advice, counsel and consensus of the radiation therapist community in the development of an

ASRT position statement establishing baccalaureate degree entry-level professional standards for radiation therapists by the year 2000."

In response, the ASRT formed a Task Force on Educational Standards for Radiation Therapists. Under the leadership of chairman Carole Sullivan, the task force began working toward establishing the baccalaureate as the entry-level standard for the profession. It first developed articulation guidelines between certificate, associate degree and baccalaureate programs that would allow students to transfer course credits from hospital-based educational programs to four-year teaching institutions.

The United States was not alone in considering the elevation of educational standards for radiation therapists; England, Australia and other countries began phasing in degree programs in the early 1990s. The United States, by contrast, seemed woefully behind. In 1990 only five of the 111 CAHEA-accredited radiation therapy programs in the United States offered baccalaureate degrees; the majority of programs still offered one-year curriculums. The number of baccalaureate programs increased to nine out of a total of 120 CAHEA-approved programs by 1993.

The Task Force on Educational Standards for Radiation Therapists continued its work through 1992, encouraging input from therapists, administrators and educators in an effort to build consensus. In 1993 the task force presented a resolution to the ASRT House of Delegates calling for all students entering radiation therapy programs in the year 2000 and afterward to complete a baccalaureate degree for entry into the profession. At the House meeting, debate centered on whether requiring a baccalaureate degree would cause undue hardship on students. In the end, however, the resolution was adopted. Sullivan hailed the action, calling it the first

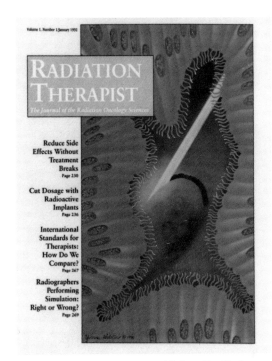

In 1992 the ASRT began publishing Radiation Therapist, *the first professional journal devoted exclusively to radiation therapists.*

step in therapists' efforts to achieve professional status.

Following approval of the elevated entry-level standard, the ASRT immediately began updating the radiation therapy curriculum. Only after the curriculum is approved and new accreditation standards are in place can the ASRT petition the Department of Labor for professional status for radiation therapists.

By June 30, 1994, almost 10,000 radiation therapists were certified by the Registry. The profession's growth had been phenomenal: the 277 radiation therapists certified in 1969 grew to 1,942 by 1979 and surged to 6,527 in 1989. The achievements the profession reached along the way were equally impressive. Radiation therapists had earned an integral position on the cancer treatment team, working alongside the radiation oncologist, oncology nurse, physicist and dosimetrist. In addition, more and more therapists were pursuing careers in education, research, department

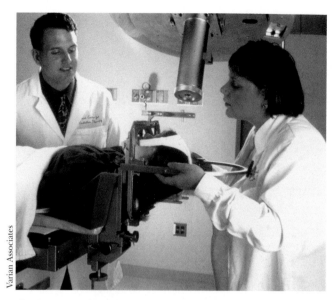

Varian Associates

Stereotactic radiotherapy is the newest form of three-dimensional conformal therapy.

administration, hyperthermia and dosimetry.

The discipline also continued its efforts to further distinguish itself from diagnostic radiology, establishing its own scope of practice in 1993 and its own code of ethics in 1994. The personnel shortage that had gripped the discipline for more than a decade lessened somewhat during the early 1990s, and salaries began to improve.

Radiation therapists traditionally were better paid than other radiologic science professionals. A 1975 ASRT survey reported average annual salaries of $11,398 for radiation therapists and $10,050 for radiographers. By 1994, according to a survey by the University of Texas Medical Branch at Galveston, radiation therapists' salaries averaged $36,023, compared with $28,497 for radiographers, $34,673 for sonographers and $35,031 for nuclear medicine technologists. The trade-off for these higher wages, however, was a high level of work-related stress. A 1993 survey showed that 95 percent of female radiation therapists rated their jobs as either "very stressful" or "somewhat stressful."

Rapidly advancing technology was responsible for at least part of the stress therapists felt. Technology continued to drive the profession, with treatment capabilities evolving at an incredible rate. Advances in the use of simulators, computed tomography and magnetic resonance imaging revolutionized treatment planning, while improvements in neutron therapy, the development of isocentric treatment and the introduction of three-dimensional "beam's eye view" systems transformed the way therapists performed their jobs.

One of the most impressive developments was conformal radiation therapy, a technology dependent on multileaf collimation and real time portal imaging. Multileaf collimators, which feature individually controlled leaves instead of a solid jaw, actually were invented in the early 1900s. It was not until the 1960s, however, that a Japanese physicist used the multileaf collimator for "conformal radiation therapy," the term he used to describe moving the leaves of the collimator to force all the radiation fields to match the irregular shape of the tumor. This technique shields healthy tissues from radiation, allowing therapists to deliver a higher dose while also decreasing the toxicity of the therapy.

In the United States, Varian Associates began developing multileaf collimators for its linear accelerators in the 1970s. The company introduced one of the newest forms of three-dimensional conformal therapy — a procedure called stereotactic radiotherapy — in the early 1990s. It uses an ultra-precise beam to irradiate tumors in the brain to within fractions of a millimeter.

The incredible complexity of these technological advances brought a new level of precision and accuracy to radiation therapy, dramatically improving cure rates for specific types of cancer. Also contributing to the improved cure rates were dramatic improvements in diagnostic radiology that enabled physicians to detect cancer earlier. Diagnostic and therapeutic radiology, working in conjunction with surgery and chemotherapy, provided patients with more treatment options and a better chance of survival. According to 1994 figures from the American Cancer Society, with early detection and aggressive treatment, 78 percent of patients with Hodgkin's disease can be cured, 90 percent of women with localized cervical cancer can be cured, 92 percent of men with localized prostate tumors can be cured and 93 percent of women with localized breast cancer can be cured.

But radiation therapy requires more than just precise technology. It also demands a high level of human caring. Because radiation therapists may interact with extremely ill patients for weeks or months at a time, compassion and sensitivity are as vital to their jobs as knowledge and expertise. Providing emotional support, education and counseling to patients and their families has become part of the radiation therapist's role, and no amount of technological sophistication will change that. In 1979 Donna K. Dunn, M.S., R.T.(T), conducted a survey to determine the factors that influenced people to choose a career in radiation therapy. The No. 1 reason, cited by 64 percent of respondents, was working with patients. When Dunn conducted the same survey 14 years later, patient contact still was the top reason cited by therapists for entering the profession.

In 1993 Dunn received the Varian Award for Achievement in Radiation Therapy. During her award lecture, she reflected on the changes radiation therapy had experienced since its establishment as a distinct discipline in the mid-1960s.

"It's incredible how much our profession has evolved in the past three decades," Dunn said. "As radiation therapists, we've witnessed the move from single hand blocked portals to multiple portals with multileaf collimating systems; from a few metropolitan radiation therapy facilities that were part of radiology departments to freestanding community-based radiation oncology departments; from superficial, orthovoltage, betatron and cobalt 60 treatment machines to dual energy linear accelerators, neutron and proton treatment machines." But through all these changes, Dunn noted, "one thing has remained constant — the very special relationship that exists between the patient and the radiation therapist."

Millions of cancer patients rely on radiation therapists and the treatments they deliver for relief from pain, confinement of malignancy and, in many cases, survival. Following a century of continual progress, radiation therapy today brings cancer patients around the world the greatest promise of all — hope.

Chapter Eleven
Multiple Identities

Radiology's first 50 years were ruled by the x-ray. This mysterious beam of light, invisible to the eye and weightless to the touch, was hailed as one of the scientific breakthroughs of the century, earned its discoverer a Nobel Prize in Physics and gave medicine a new way to diagnose injury. From 1895 to 1945, the x-ray and radiology were synonymous: radiology meant x-rays.

But technology never rests, and during the second half of radiology's first century, radiology's family tree gradually sprouted new branches. Scientists developed increasingly sophisticated diagnostic imaging techniques that used high-frequency sound waves, radio waves and magnetic waves instead of x-rays. Nuclear medicine emerged from new radiopharmaceuticals, computers transformed the radiology department, and dedicated x-ray equipment was developed for mammographic examinations. Technological advances meant that radiation was being used not only to find cancer, but increasingly to treat it. Interventional radiology procedures were developed to guide miniature instruments through the human body, reducing the pain and cost associated with surgery.

Radiology, once based on the imaging capabilities of the x-ray alone, expanded to encompass diagnostic, therapeutic and interventional medicine.

With this rapid explosion of technology, it became impossible for radiologists and radiologic technologists to achieve clinical expertise in every discipline. Technologists began to specialize in radiography, mammography, magnetic resonance imaging, computed tomography, cardiovascular-interventional technology, nuclear medicine, radiation therapy or sonography. Others moved into hospital and clinic management or the higher ranks of academia. Radiologic technology — the profession that began as a cohesive group of health care workers linked by their use of the x-ray — started to splinter into specialties.

As these new technologies, disciplines and interests emerged within the radiologic sciences, it was inevitable that specialty organizations arise to meet their needs. New special-purpose associations sprouted up outside the ASRT. Interestingly, the phenomenon struck repeatedly in a narrow time frame. In the late 1960s and early '70s, a number of technologist groups recognized a common need for separate identities and specialized education services.

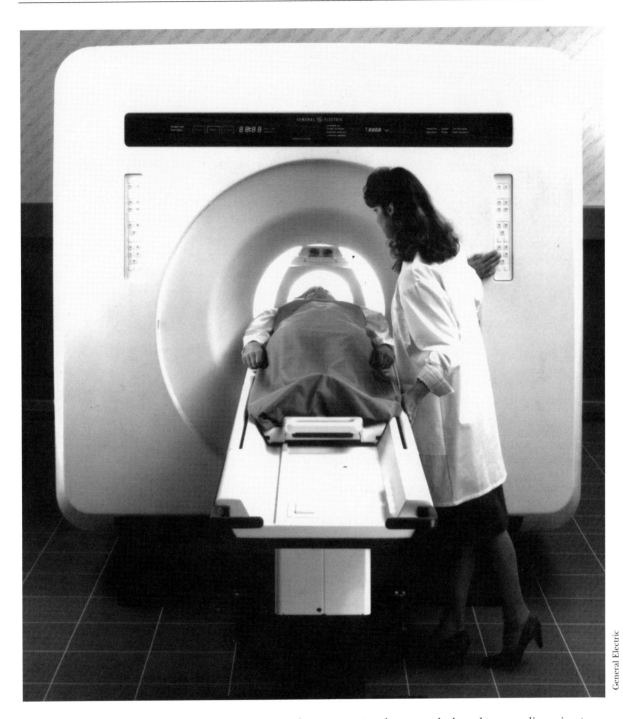

General Electric

As the first diagnostic technique to unite computers and x-rays, computed tomography brought a new dimension to medical imaging in 1972. Early units were capable of scanning only the brain. Today's sophisticated CT scanners are used for whole-body scanning and to guide needle biopsies and evaluate cancers. The ARRT began administering certification exams in CT in 1995.

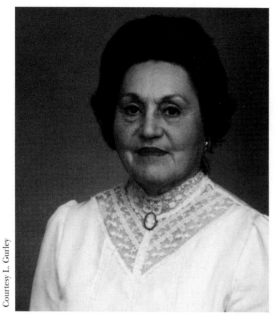

Laverne Gurley began advocating in-service education for radiologic technologists in the late 1960s.

The first of these was the Association of University Radiologic Technologists (AURT). Longtime ASRT loyalist Laverne Gurley, Ph.D., R.T.(R)(N)(T), FASRT, helped found the first independent technologist educators group because, as she said, "There was nothing else available." In 1967, 26 educators from colleges and universities throughout the country met in St. Louis to discuss how they could best establish radiologic technology as an academic career. A constitution adopted by the charter members set a three-fold purpose:

- To encourage the exchange of teaching concepts and curricula and establish minimum standards for teaching radiologic technology at the certificate, diploma, associate and baccalaureate levels.
- To stimulate an interest in academic radiologic technology as a career.
- To advance radiologic technology as an allied health science by encouraging members to conduct research and write technical papers.

Interestingly enough, the new organization immediately faced an old problem. At the time, continuing education for technologists was not encouraged. In 1969 Gurley, a long-time advocate of in-service education, presented the first lecture on this subject at the AURT annual meeting. She said that when she finished, "A radiologist came up to me and asked, 'How does your boss feel about you being involved with in-service education?'" The perception that a little knowledge is a dangerous thing "was indelibly stamped in the mind of every physician in the country," she added.

But changes in the 1970s set the stage for new attitudes about educational standards. Nurses were required by the American Hospital Association (AHA) to attend in-service education for hospitals to maintain their accreditation. Hospital administrators regarded in-service education in the nursing profession as a sound investment and many employed in-service education directors on the nursing staff.

This led Gurley and other radiologic technology educators to petition the AHA, the Association of Schools of Allied Health Professionals (ASAHP) and others to set similar requirements for technologists. "Why do you require it for nurses and you don't require it for us? Our technology is changing much more rapidly than theirs is," said Gurley, who at the time worked at the University of Tennessee College of Medicine.

Much like earlier battles waged by the ASRT for support from the radiologist community and the AMA, changes were slow in coming for the AURT. But Gurley pressed forward, undeterred. In 1969 she published in ASRT's *Radiologic Technology* what is probably the first article on in-service education for technologists. Citing lack of uniformity in educational programs throughout the country, Gurley stated: "While in-service education may be firmly established in many professions, it is in its infancy in radiologic technology. This has been a great failing in our profession."

The rapid growth and acceptance of community colleges also contributed to change. At first animosity existed between the new institutions and what some considered the college and university "elitists." But once the community college system was in place, the AURT set out to expand and develop curricula and methods of program evaluation. "At that time, even the university programs weren't degree programs. Most programs were hospital certificate programs," Gurley said.

As radiologic technologists struggled to find their place in academia, other career paths opened in unfamiliar territory. Even in the late 1960s, radiologists were managing day-to-day operations in radiology departments in most hospitals across the country. But the paperwork load, in the form of Medicare and Medicaid reimbursement claims and a multitude of other administrative hoops, became unbearable for professionals whose real interest was in practicing medicine. Into the breach stepped the technologist.

In many cases, the chief technologist assumed the administrator role. But depending upon the institution's philosophy, any number of other health care specialists, as well as business managers, were offered the radiology administrator position. From the hospital and private practice venues two different yet similar groups of radiology administrators emerged.

In 1968 a group of administrators, most of whom worked in the private practice setting, formed the Radiology Business Management Association (RBMA). These managers faced many of the same challenges as hospital department administrators, but they did not have to contend with the problems that went with large staffs typical of hospitals or the internal administrative requirements.

At the time, the RBMA did not accept hospital administrators into its ranks. As a result, in 1973 the American Hospital Radiology Administrators (AHRA) was formed by Hal Magida, Edward Cohen, Robert Wagner and Tammy Waldhauser. They were joined by Howard Beam, Marion O'Toole and Michael Thomas, who expanded the geographical scope of the fledgling organization. Spearheading a survey of hospital administrators nationwide, Magida, who served as the AHRA's founding force and first president, found an odd mix of pharmacists, physicists, technologists, nurses, doctors and business managers working in clinical management.

Although the hospital administrative functions of a radiology department could be and often were handled by a chief technologist, it often detracted from the "hands-on" aspects of the technologist's training. AHRA member Louise Broadley, FAHRA, who received her technologist training in the Navy during the 1940s and later served as administrator of radiological services at N.Y. Medical College, noted: "Ten years ago I would have said that there is a definite advantage in having a technologist as a radiology administrator. I no longer think that. Nowadays, administrators have quality assurance people to oversee the imaging aspect."

It was difficult to choose a name because we didn't want to get involved with the technician-technologist controversy that was going on at the time...

This became especially true for large urban facilities where radiology departments were destined to become big business, dealing with multimillion dollar budgets, complex labor negotiations, labyrinthine regulatory management and documentation. But in rural hospitals it remained more common to find radiology administrators whose function was both chief technologist and business manager.

In-service educators and radiology administrators were just the beginning of the specialized splinter groups. During a 1969 annual meeting of the American Institute of Ultrasound in Medicine (AIUM), in Winnipeg, Canada, six technical specialists, including Joan P. Baker, M.S.R., RDMS, Marilyn Ball, Margaret Byrne, James Dennon, Raylene Husak and L.E. Schnitzer, met and decided it was time to form an association for technologists performing ultrasound procedures.

While the AIUM board of directors did not oppose the formation of the technologist society, the majority believed the technologists were wasting their time and the action was premature. The technologists forged ahead, and at the AIUM's 1970 annual meeting in Cleveland, Ohio, the American Society of Ultrasound Technical Specialists (ASUTS) was chartered. "It was difficult to choose a name because we didn't want to get involved with the technician-technologist controversy that was going on at the time," Baker said.

In a chapter on the history of diagnostic ultrasound for a Smithsonian Institution exhibit, Baker wrote, "The early officers of ASUTS had a particular commonality: They were all dedicated teachers who had been involved in the early, rapid growth of this new modality. All were acutely aware of the serious shortage of technical specialists — but more importantly, they understood that the future of ultrasound was dependent upon the ability of the field to provide qualified manpower."

During the next decade, the technical specialist group established its own annual meeting, its own registry and a separate educational accreditation body. The group succeeded in having the AMA officially recognize its discipline as "diagnostic ultrasound technology," and established executive offices in Dallas. The "technical specialists" became "sonographers" in 1974, and in 1980 ASUTS changed its name to what it is known as today — the Society of Diagnostic Medical Sonogra-

phers (SDMS).

Unlike their sonographer colleagues, technologists in nuclear medicine who sought to form their own organization never split from their fostering physician organization. The Board of the Society of Nuclear Medicine (SNM) early on recognized the need to serve its technologist members, establishing a Committee on Nuclear Medicine Technologists, chaired by Ervin Kaplan, M.D., of Chicago.

As early as 1966, a group of nuclear medicine technologists in Houston petitioned for formal affiliation with SNM. The group's leader, Gary Wood, worked with SNM's Thomas P. Haynie, M.D., and the SNM's Southwest Chapter to include technologists in chapter bylaws.

By 1969 Haynie requested a stronger voice for technologists in nuclear medicine's professional society. In a letter to SNM President-elect George Taplin, M.D., Haynie proposed developing a technologist section with SNM, allowing for the election of its own officers and separate meetings to coincide with those of the main society. Less than three weeks later, SNM President C. Craig Harris, Ph.D., addressed the issue in his report to the board of trustees, suggesting the chapter representation of technologists be expanded to a different kind of national level representation.

In 1970 the trustees approved revised bylaws proposed by Wood and Haynie that created the Technologist Section, which held its first business meeting in 1971. Like most of its contemporary organizations, the SNM Technologist Section devoted much of its energies to education. This effort led to the creation of its own scholarly journal, the Nuclear Medicine Technology Certification Board (NMTCB) and the Verification of Involvement in Continuing Education program (VOICE).

The special purpose organizations did not totally exist without input and cooperation

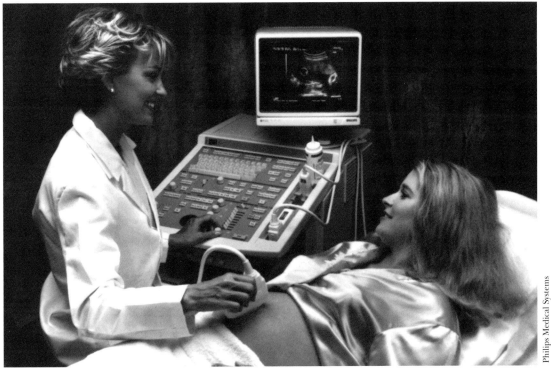

Philips Medical Systems

Ultrasound's growth as an imaging modality spawned the formation of the American Society of Ultrasound Technical Specialists in 1970. The organization changed its name in 1980 to the Society of Diagnostic Medical Sonographers.

from the ASRT. The Society had more than 50 years of hard-earned experience to offer from its relentless efforts in striving for educational consistency in all radiologic science professions. Committees often exchanged ideas and discussed problems common to the organizations.

As the Society celebrated its 60th anniversary in 1980, many of the technologists who had actively participated during the formative years recognized — with no small amount of chagrin — that their organization had grown beyond the "family." The Society itself began to restructure, bending to the demands of the time. Regional directors were installed as a result of the growing affiliate membership. A professional lobbyist guarded the ASRT's growing legislative interests in Washington, D.C. The old guard made way for a new generation.

Whether or not history will judge the

decade of the 1980s with kindness remains to be seen, but it was as turbulent in its own right as those of the war years or of the technological growth of the 1960s. The 1980s had their own peculiarities. American business changed dramatically. Mass, instantaneous communication broadened horizons. A global consciousness emerged. Of most significance, however, was the way American business thought about profit and the bottom line. Quality became a buzzword. Unemployment soared. Political gridlock was the norm. Medical care costs took on a life of their own. Technology grew more important than technique.

For the radiologic technologist — and the ASRT — maintaining a cohesive front through those times was as difficult a task as any the Society had faced. Diversity became even more prominent. Fortunately for the ASRT, which stood firm on its primary focus of education, passage through this era cemented the Society's goals for the future. Other groups were still searching for their rightful place.

The AURT, for example, underwent a name change in 1984, becoming the Association of Educators in Radiological Sciences (AERS) to reflect the organization's growing membership in all imaging modalities and radiation therapy. At that time, the association's active members were certified by the ARRT, the newly formed American Registry of Diagnostic Medical Sonography or the Nuclear Medicine Technologists Certifying Board. Members of the AERS were employed as full- or part-time educators in nationally certified programs or employed with educational responsibilities in the radiologic sciences. By 1995 AERS membership grew to more than 900, with the association's headquarters located in Oak Brook, Ill.

Shortly after the AERS began, more and more hospitals approached colleges and universities to take over their radiography education programs. The medical facilities wanted out of the education business to focus their efforts on patient care. Changes in technology and educational regulation by the government were leaving them hard-pressed to keep current.

This propelled hospital program directors into the realm of post-secondary education, but many found themselves ill prepared to handle the details of funding, curriculum development, state and federal regulations and the many academic protocols of the university environment.

In 1975 representatives from 12 Western U.S. colleges and universities formed the Western Intercollegiate Consortium on Education in Radiologic Technology (WICERT). The founders sought to improve the quality of college-level radiologic technology by providing a network for radiologic science educa-

tors who found themselves newcomers to the college and university setting.

The consortium's boundaries included the seven Western states of California, Oregon, Washington, Idaho, Utah, Wyoming and Nevada. WICERT patterned its institutional membership structure after the Western Institutional Consortium for Nursing Education and the Association of Schools of Allied Health Professions.

From the outset, technically based programs faced an uphill battle to achieve credibility and recognition in the university arena. Jane Van Valkenburg, Ph.D., R.T.(R)(N), FASRT, WICERT's first vice president, noted, "Some academicians felt we were contaminating their territory, and we received little help from colleagues in other university departments, especially when it came to federal funding. We were all foundering at first." The group persisted, maintaining an informal philosophy that promoted the need for research and sharing instructional methodologies.

This became evident during the group's annual meetings, which were characterized by small discussion groups in which members exchanged information, sought solutions to common problems and developed long-lasting relationships with fellow radiologic technology educators.

In the coming years, the organization's accomplishments would include standardizing course content to facilitate the transfer of credits among member institutions, publishing the book *Principles and Practices of the College-based Radiologic Science Program*, developing curricula for health administration, health education, advanced radiography, mammography and quality assurance, and developing student admission criteria.

In 1991 a name change to the Association of Collegiate Educators in Radiologic Technology (ACERT) recognized the organization's expanding geographic membership

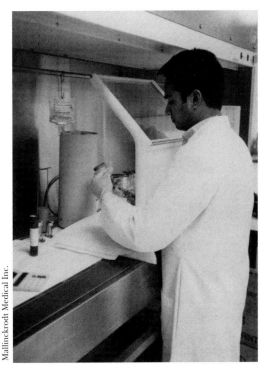

An estimated 12 million nuclear medicine proce-dures are performed annually in the United States.

and evolution to include all imaging and therapeutic disciplines. By 1995 ACERT counted nearly 40 member institutions and associate members in states well beyond its original Western borders. The non-profit educational organization today maintains its headquarters at Weber State University in Ogden, Utah.

Similar to the progress enjoyed by the educators, radiology administrators also savored successes. In 1986 the AHRA, reacting to the changing nature of U.S. health care, changed its guidelines and its name to the American Healthcare Radiology Administrators to include members from freestanding imaging centers.

The association, headquartered in Sudbury, Mass., swelled in membership from its few founders to nearly 4,000 in 1995. Its diverse membership helped guide the association in its dealings with other radiology organizations. For example, in 1987 AHRA organized the Summit on Manpower, an 18-member coali-

tion of national health care organizations whose overall goal was to reduce the personnel shortage in medical imaging and radiation therapy. Among the key members of the Summit, besides the ASRT, were the SDMS (with a membership of more than 10,000) and the SNM/TS (more than 6,500 members strong in 1995). The Summit successfully saw a quick turnaround in the radiology employment situation and moved on to tackle other, larger issues, such as health care reform.

Just as the need for advanced education and radiology administration gave rise to these groups, technological innovations continued to bring other groups together. One such technology was magnetic resonance imaging (MRI), based upon the principle that certain nuclei have a magnetic moment. Although this concept was first postulated in the 1920s, it was not until the 1940s that scientists were able to demonstrate the effect.

By 1977 researchers built the first prototype and performed the first human scan. By the end of the 1970s, MRI scanners were available commercially, and since then MR medical applications have expanded nearly exponentially. Early on, however, hospital radiology departments scrambled to find personnel who could perform the new examination. Quite often they turned to radiologic technologists already experienced in computed tomography, because both CT and MRI require extensive knowledge of cross-sectional anatomy. Later, some of these technologists chose to specialize in MRI.

The technologists working in MRI at its infancy could not have imagined all the technical advances and new applications that would unfold. Through the mid-1980s MRI was used mainly for neuroradiology and imaging the musculoskeletal system. By the early 1990s its medical applications surged into MR angiography, functional MR and cardiac MR.

In search of continuing education in this

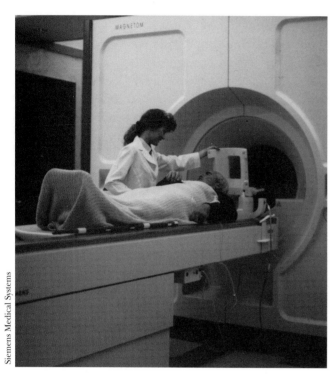

Siemens Medical Systems

Introduced in the late 1970s, magnetic resonance imaging now is being used in angiography, perfusion imaging and functional imaging. The ARRT began administering certification exams in MRI in 1995.

fast-paced science, MRI technologists began attending annual meetings of the Society of Magnetic Resonance in Medicine (SMRM) and the Society for Magnetic Resonance Imaging (SMRI). The SMRM, established in 1980 by physicians and scientists, was created to promote research in magnetic resonance in the medical sciences. The SMRI was chartered in 1982 by clinical and basic scientists devoted to researching magnetic resonance techniques in medicine, with emphasis on imaging. The annual educational conferences of both organizations were designed to forge a link between the raw science of magnetic resonance and its clinical applications in diagnostic imaging.

As technologist attendance grew at their annual conferences, the SMRM and SMRI realized by the mid-1980s that they needed to offer education sessions specific to technolo-

gists. The response to those new educational sessions was overwhelming, with hundreds of MRI technologists traveling thousands of miles to attend.

Bill Faulkner, R.T.(R), recalls, "The desire for education was what motivated these technologists. They were trying to keep up with the technology. MRI had grown phenomenally since its first clinical use, and technologists were starved for education. The SMRM and SMRI meetings were about the only place you could get it. Eventually, you began seeing the same technologists at both conferences. By 1990 a group of us began talking about forming our own technologist section."

SMRM and SMRI supported the idea, and at the 1991 RSNA meeting in Chicago, a committee of radiologists, physicists and technologists from both groups gathered to draft the articles of cooperation for the combined Section for Magnetic Resonance Technologists (SMRT). Faulkner was elected president of the Section by its 300 members. By 1995 SMRT's membership ballooned to more than 1,000.

The formation of the technologist section was driven solely by the need to keep pace with the rapid evolution of the technology. According to Faulkner, "Because the quality of an MR image is very dependent on the skills of the technologist, the SMRM and SMRI recognized the importance of providing continuing education through an organization that was geared specifically toward technologists."

The technologist section set up business operations in Berkeley, Calif., where the SMRM office was located. Its board of directors consisted of an equal number of SMRT, SMRM and SMRI officers.

By 1992 SMRT had firmly established itself as a provider of MR technologist education. It began publishing a quarterly newsletter and hosting its own annual meeting, featuring clinical plenary symposia and papers and posters presented by technologists. The SMRT also sponsored six regional educational seminars annually for the benefit of technologists who could not attend the annual meeting. On Jan. 1, 1994, the SMRM and SMRI merged to form the Society for Magnetic Resonance (SMR), representing more than 3,600 physicians, physicists, engineers and biochemists. The SMRT became an affiliated section of the new society, welcoming technologists working in magnetic resonance at the clinical or research level to join its ranks.

During this period of reinvention when so many specialty associations formed, the ASRT was far from stagnant. While the specialty associations that emerged during the 1960s, '70s and '80s focused on meeting the needs of specific groups of technologists, the ASRT continued working on behalf of the profession as a whole. The Society took a more active role in politics, curriculum development and continuing education. It established positive working relationships with many of the new associations and worked closer than ever with the ARRT and JRCERT.

By representing all radiologic technologists, no matter what their discipline or interest, the Society maintained its leadership position in the radiologic sciences. The foresight and action of ASRT leaders and members helped determine the direction of the entire radiologic technology profession.

Chapter Twelve

New Beginnings

The profession entered its eighth decade with an impressive series of wins under its belt. The 1981 passage of the Radiation Health and Safety Act, in particular, graphically illustrated the full reach of the ASRT and the unwavering determination of its leaders and members. The toll this victory took on the Society, however, rapidly became apparent. Its 13-year battle for licensure, combined with skyrocketing national inflation rates and the high cost of doing business in Chicago, nearly drained ASRT coffers. Almost overnight, the Society was forced to turn its attention from fighting professional battles to fighting for its own survival.

The crisis was real, with bankruptcy looming unless the Society dramatically improved its financial condition. During 1980 ASRT pared its operating budget by more than $70,000. Every expense was trimmed, from postage to printing, and the already lean ASRT office staff was reduced from 17 to 14. Although these measures helped, the Society remained in jeopardy. With cash resources rapidly dwindling, the ASRT was five months from closing its doors in the summer of 1981. It was obvious that budget cuts alone weren't enough to stop the financial drain.

The only thing that could save the Society was an increase in membership dues. Annual dues stood at $30 in 1981, unchanged since 1975 despite a 53 percent increase in the cost of doing business. Two attempts in 1980 to raise dues by a mere $10 to keep pace with inflation were defeated by the members, an indication that they recognized neither the depth of the Society's financial crisis nor the true value of their ASRT membership. Research showed it cost the ASRT nearly $60 to provide services to each member each year, only half of which was covered by membership dues.

Faced with the grim possibility of shutting down the 60-year-old Society, the ASRT Board of Directors recommended a 100 percent dues increase at its mid-year meeting in December 1980. The $30 increase would bring annual dues to $60 — closer to the actual cost of servicing each member, yet one of the lowest rates for a professional health care organization at the time. The Board's recommendation meant nothing, however, unless the membership approved the dues increase at the 1981 Annual Conference.

"We are now at the point where further cutbacks are not the answer," Executive Director Ward Keller, R.T.(R), told the Society's 20,000 members in mid-1981, noting that

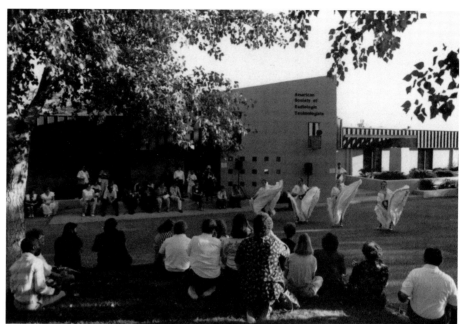

In 1991 the ASRT sponsored the ISRRT Conference of the Americas in conjunction with the ASRT Annual Conference in Albuquerque, N.M. The honors reception held at the Society's office featured an international theme.

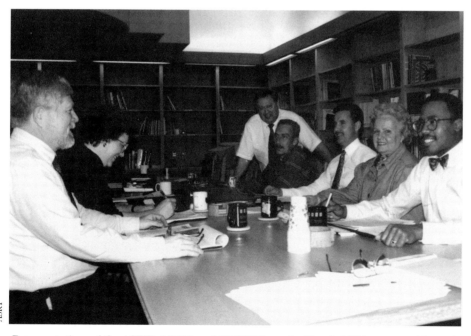

Representatives of the ASRT, ARRT and JRCERT met in March 1994 to set specific goals to strengthen the profession. From left are Darrell McKay, Jan Sisler and ASRT Chief Executive Officer Ward Keller, representing the ASRT; Sal Martino and ARRT Executive Director Jerry Reid, representing the Registry; and JRCERT Executive Director Marilyn Fay and Michael Ward, representing the JRCERT.

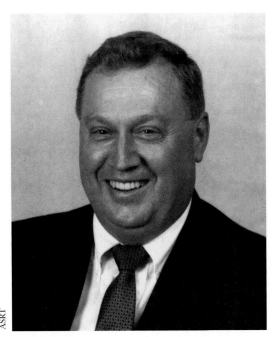

Ward Keller, ASRT chief executive officer.

additional budget reductions would affect traditional member services and undercut the very reason for the Society's existence. "The reality exists that without this dues increase, ASRT will cease operations this year. We are at a critical turning point."

Despite a full agenda of lectures, workshops and business meetings, the dues increase was the main topic of conversation at the 1981 ASRT Annual Conference in Salt Lake City, July 10-16. Ward Keller, ASRT President Marilyn Holland, R.T.(R), and other Society officers spent much of the conference's first few days addressing the members in attendance, asking them to understand the Society's dire financial situation and encouraging them to vote in favor of the dues increase.

Tension mounted as the day of the vote approached. When Marilyn Holland convened the Society's July 14 business meeting, a member motioned from the floor for an immediate vote on the $30 dues increase. Holland heard scattered murmurs through the crowd, and then Sergeant-at-Arms Al

Robinson, R.T.(R), rose and made a motion that the dues increase pass with unanimous approval. This meant an objection from just one member could defeat the measure.

From the podium, Holland repeated Robinson's request for unanimous approval of the dues increase and asked if there were any objections. After a moment of silence, Holland gazed out over the assembly and repeated her question. A complete stillness again filled the room, broken only when Holland dropped her gavel and announced the unanimous approval of the dues increase from the assembly in Salt Lake City. The crowd rose to its feet, greeting the announcement with thunderous applause. Members' pledge of support for their Society was reinvigorating, and a feeling of camaraderie swept through the crowd and permeated the remainder of the conference.

The dues increase went into effect Nov. 1, 1981, pulling the ASRT back from the edge of financial collapse. Vowing they would never again brush so close to disaster, Society leaders immediately began working on a plan to ensure long-term financial stability for the organization. Top on their list was a possible relocation of the ASRT executive offices.

Relocation first had come into consideration in the late 1970s, when rent and utilities for the ASRT's Chicago office became the organization's single largest expense. Chicago was the fifth most expensive city in the world in which to operate a business, and downtown office rents jumped an average 130 percent between 1978 and 1982. Combined, ASRT's rent and utility bills rose from $58,900 in 1978 to $85,600 in 1982 and were expected to increase to $110,000 or higher in 1983. Even at those prices, the ASRT was on the low end of the rent scale for downtown Chicago.

The thousands spent on rent left no money for investments or to establish equity or collateral for even a short-term loan. Rising inflation

The Evolving Curriculum

The ASRT professional curricula establish which subjects should be taught in radiography and radiation therapy programs to adequately educate technologists. Revisions to the curriculum through the years reflected changes not only in the profession, but in American culture in general. For example, the "ethics" unit in the 1960 radiography curriculum guide concentrated on topics such as grooming, posture, cleanliness, courtesy and cooperation. By 1983, the ethics unit had evolved to focus on issues such as the radiographer's scope of practice, limits of responsibility, legal liability and informed consent.

The profession's first curriculum guide was published by the ASXT in 1952. Titled "The Basic Curriculum and Teacher's Syllabus in X-Ray Technology," the guide described a 200-hour, one-year program of study. It was a first step in standardizing radiography education and enjoyed widespread popularity among educational program directors.

As technology advanced, the radiography curriculum grew to incorporate new equipment, techniques and teaching methods. In 1960 the curriculum was revised to a 400-hour, two-year program of study. Because it was developed during the Cold War era, this version of the curriculum included a unit on civil defense. More than 50 educators collaborated with the ASXT to revise the document, using a two-year curriculum published by the Catholic Hospital Association as a guide.

Perhaps the most extensive revision of the curriculum guide began in 1971, when ASRT President Leslie Wilson appointed Ward Keller, R.T.(R), to chair a task force to rewrite the document. Starting almost from scratch, the task force produced a curriculum guide that covered anatomy, pathology, medical terminology, radiographic film processing and evaluation, patient care, imaging techniques, exposure principles, radiographic principles, radiologic physics, radiation protection and radiation biology. It was published in September 1976.

For the 1983 revision of the radiography curriculum guide, units were added on professional development, quality assurance and computer literacy. By 1993, the range of topics had grown to include digital radiology, MRI hardware and software, pharmacology and patient scheduling systems.

Throughout its history, the radiography curriculum has continually expanded to embrace changes in society and advances in the radiologic sciences. It is one of the profession's best examples of a living document.

—*Ceela McElveny*

rates during the late 1970s made purchasing property a serious consideration, yet the ASRT owned no assets beyond a few typewriters and desks. More than any other factor, its Chicago location seemed to limit the future welfare and expansion of the Society.

In 1980 the Board of Directors appointed a Task Force on Relocation to make recommendations about whether to move the office, and if so, where. The task force's findings, made public at the 1982 Annual Conference, reached the unavoidable conclusion that to save money and build for the future, the ASRT needed to leave Chicago. The news took many members by surprise. Chicago was home to nearly 100 medical organizations, including the American Medical Association, the Radiological Society of North America

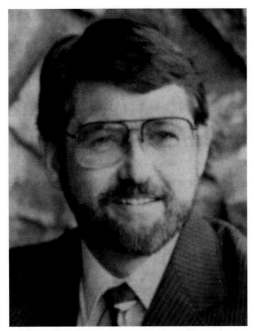

James A. Mom, ASRT president 1982-83.

and the Joint Review Committee on Education in Radiologic Technology. The ASRT's executive office had been located in Chicago only since 1968, but its ties to the Windy City ran deep: Ed Jerman founded the Society at the Morrison Hotel in Chicago on Oct. 25, 1920, and members met annually in the city until 1930.

The Board of Directors and the Task Force on Relocation, however, agreed that the Society could no longer justify the expense of a downtown Chicago address. The Society conducted most of its business with other Chicago medical associations by mail, with the few face-to-face meetings taking place at the associations' various annual conferences instead of in their offices. Annual meetings rarely took place in Chicago, and the cost to send executives to such meetings was insignificant compared to the savings represented by moving ASRT to a less expensive city.

Soon, the search was on for a new home for the Society. Suggestions from members poured in, with many urging the ASRT to relocate to a Chicago suburb such as Oak

Brook or Glen Ellyn. The Board of Directors, however, found that the predicted savings of $10,000 to $20,000 per year "would not be appreciable enough to justify the move" to the suburbs. Other members asked the Board to consider moving the office to Washington, D.C., to gain easy access to the halls of Congress. The Board briefly considered this possibility until it discovered that office rents in the District of Columbia rivaled those of downtown Chicago. In addition, a professional lobbyist had been contracted to perform most of the Society's work on Capitol Hill, leaving little reason to locate the entire business office there.

The Task Force on Relocation drew up a list of 12 cities around the country and spent much of 1982 gathering data about each prospective site, focusing on everything from local property values to airline service. The Society planned to use industrial development bonds, which helped businesses finance property with a low-interest loan, to purchase its own office building. With these bonds, the ASRT finally would be able to own property and develop equity for the Society's future.

By the end of the year, the task force's list had been narrowed to three cities that offered industrial development bonds: Albuquerque, N.M.; Nashville, Tenn.; and Austin, Texas. Task force members visited each of the candidate cities, meeting with local officials, school boards, real estate agents, land developers and business leaders and touring business and residential properties. Their investigation showed that Austin's cost of living was about the same as the Chicago suburbs, representing little savings to ASRT. This narrowed the choice to Nashville or Albuquerque. Because relocation costs and other economic considerations were virtually equal for both cities, the task force reached a tie vote and could not make a final recommendation to the Board of Directors.

The War Waged For Women

"**I** am here to embark with you on one of the most important missions the health care community has ever waged for American women. It is a mission mandated by Congress and demanded by our professional standards. It is the right thing to do," said U.S. Food and Drug Administration Commissioner David A. Kessler, M.D., announcing the establishment of the Mammography Quality Standards Act of 1992. MQSA marked the first time the federal government spread its regulatory wings to institute comprehensive quality control standards in the diagnostic imaging profession.

The closest the federal government came to establishing extensive quality control regulations for radiologic procedures was the Radiation Health and Safety Act of 1981, which called for state certification of any individual who performed health care procedures that used ionizing radiation. President Ronald Reagan, by executive order, changed the Act's mandatory standards to voluntary guidelines.

Many believe the catalyst for MQSA came from the results of a 1985 study on mammography by the FDA. The study was one of many under the heading National Evaluation of X-Ray Trends (NEXT). The FDA reported a wide range of equipment, dose and image quality problems in mammography.

A year following the FDA's report, the American College of Radiology established its Mammography Accreditation Program and began accrediting sites in 1987. Although well received, the accreditation program was strictly voluntary. The ACR

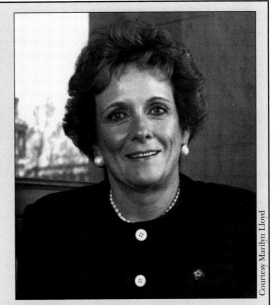

Rep. Marilyn Lloyd was instrumental in developing the Mammography Quality Standards Act. Lloyd was diagnosed with breast cancer in 1991.

estimated that by 1993 approximately 65 percent of mammography sites were accredited. "The ACR is not a regulatory body," said Marie Zinninger, assistant executive director of the ACR. "We can't force radiology departments into accreditation. That, only the government can do."

Realizing they could only get so far with voluntary accreditation, breast cancer organizations turned to government legislation and the media.

Much of the urgency in improving the diagnosis and treatment of breast cancers stemmed from the grim and steady rise in the incidence of the disease — from 89,000 in 1975, or one in 15 women contracting breast cancer during their lifetime, to 180,000 in 1994, or one in eight contracting breast cancer. By 1991 breast cancer became the leading cause of death for American women between the ages of 15 and 54.

The most effective means of diagnosis

was the dedicated mammography unit, designed specifically to detect breast cancer. If caught early, the five-year survival rate for breast cancer was 94 percent. The American Cancer Society launched a campaign to create awareness of the benefits of early mammography screening. The ACS's success was obvious as press releases spilled into news reports. Back-to-back investigative media reports hammered mammography's patchwork standards and quality control.

Using the FDA's NEXT study and the media frenzy over mammography standards as a foothold, lobbying groups pushed women's health issues, especially breast cancer, to the forefront of the Congressional agenda. The group's efforts gained strong support from former First Ladies and Congresswomen who had contracted breast cancer.

A strong advocate of mammography legislation, Rep. Marilyn Lloyd, D-Tenn., in a great twist of irony was diagnosed with breast cancer in June 1991. Lloyd had no history of breast cancer in her family and had received a clean bill of health from a mammogram a year before. "If I had waited until next year to have another mammogram, it would have been too late for me," she told Congressional colleagues. Eight days after a radical mastectomy, she returned to work to again lead the fight for breast cancer legislation. Her efforts and personal experience paid off.

Lloyd and other legislators built on the 1990 Omnibus Budget Reconciliation Act that provided coverage for breast cancer screening for Medicare-eligible women. The legislation also required Medicare to withhold reimbursement for procedures unless technologists, radiologists and physicists were licensed or certified and dedicated mammography equipment was being used, along with a number of quality control procedures. These were the strictest set of reimbursement requirements in radiology.

Lloyd and Rep. Patricia Schroeder, D-Colo., introduced the Breast Cancer Screening Safety Act of 1991, which evolved into the Mammography Quality Standards Act. MQSA was signed into law by President George Bush on Oct. 27, 1992, and was largely based on the ACR's Mammography Accreditation Program.

Under MQSA rules, federal and state inspectors were to conduct annual on-site inspections of the country's more than 11,000 mammography sites to ensure that they met quality assurance standards. The FDA trained between 250 and 300 inspectors to perform this mammoth task, which began Oct. 1, 1994. Inspectors were specially trained to evaluate each facility's image quality, review the qualifications of its personnel and the performance of its equipment, and assess its quality assurance and control programs. If the mammography facilities did not meet the accreditation standards, they would be shut down. By mid-1995, the ACR and the states of Arkansas, California and Iowa had been approved by the FDA as accrediting bodies.

Because the federal government had intervened so little in the practice of radiology, many practitioners were shocked when Congress enacted MQSA. If Congress had to legislate a modality, why not chest radiography, many asked? After all, lung cancer was the number one killer of women and men in 1994, taking 59,000 female and 94,000 male lives and typically diagnosed by a chest x-ray. Many believed the government's actions were somewhat arbitrary, elevating the importance of accuracy in mammography over radiography or other radiology disciplines where the need for quality control was equally important.

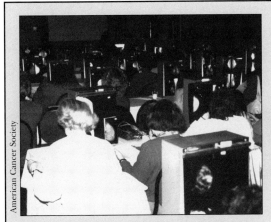

Hundreds of radiologic technologists attended a film evaluation workshop as part of an American Cancer Society mammography conference in 1995.

But unlike lung cancer, typically the product of cigarette smoking, breast cancer strikes randomly. Its victims many times share no commonalities. Experts have tried to ascribe the disease to such high-risk categories as age, family history, late or no pregnancies, late menopause and early menarche. But even the experts are befuddled by breast cancer's seemingly haphazard choice of victims, striking fear among women. That panic, fueled by the women's movement and new attention being paid to women's health issues, ultimately led to the passage of MQSA.

Many saw mammography legislation as government interference, bringing more bureaucracy and regulations than necessary. "There were always those institutions that thought they were practicing good mammography, and they felt they didn't need ACR accreditation," said the ACR's Zinninger. "The ones who knew they weren't practicing good mammography didn't apply for accreditation. So in that sense, the only way to make everyone comply was through government regulations."

Other than mammography, all radiologic science disciplines operate under voluntary accreditation standards. Due to lack of standardization in these disciplines, many experts believe it's only a matter of time before the government steps in to regulate them as well.

— Marla Poteet

But in early 1983, task force members learned that although Nashville honored industrial development bonds, it charged an "in lieu" tax on properties financed with them. The tax would add up to more than $250,000 over the life of the revenue bond. In Albuquerque, by contrast, buildings financed with development bonds were exempt from real estate and property taxes for the duration of the bond. This news ended the stalemate, and the task force recommended to the Board of Directors that the Society relocate its office to a purchased site in Albuquerque. It estimated that the ASRT would spend $1.59 million to remain in Chicago for the next 10 years, compared with $1.2 million if it moved to Nashville and $970,000 if it operated from Albuquerque. Plus, by moving to Albuquerque, the ASRT could own property for the first time.

The Board accepted the task force's recommendation on Feb. 11, 1983. Ward Keller, ASRT President James A. Mom, R.T.(R), and John Schloss, R.T.(R), were directed to find a site and finalize the relocation. They applied for an industrial development bond, which was granted immediate approval by the Albuquerque City Council, and applied for funding from a local bank.

Following announcement of the decision, James Mom addressed the membership's uneasiness about relocating the ASRT office to Albuquerque. The primary concern was that the recent dues increase was financing the move. He adamantly denied the rumor. "The dues increase was absolutely necessary

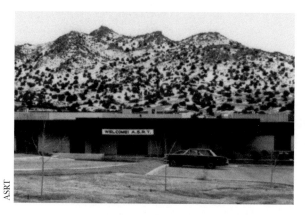
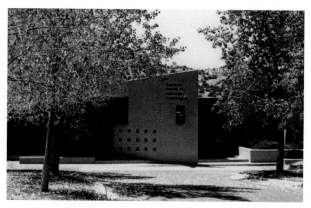

In 1984 the ASRT relocated its office from Chicago to the foothills of the Sandia Mountains in Albuquerque, N.M. Cottonwood saplings were planted in front of the building. By 1995 the building had undergone extensive renovation and the cottonwoods were more than 30 feet tall.

to save ASRT from a certain bankruptcy," said Mom. "The relocation is intended to reduce the future operating expenses of the Society and to develop equity for the future."

But if the money didn't come from the dues increase, how could ASRT afford to relocate? The Board based the Society's 1983 budget on an anticipated 40 percent membership decrease as a result of higher dues. The actual drop was only 25 percent, to about 15,000, leaving enough funds to move without jeopardizing ASRT's financial status.

Still, many members questioned the thoroughness of the Board's investigation. Mom responded again, noting that the Board of Directors "spent nearly three years making this decision and would not take the risk of making such a drastic, potentially expensive move without carefully evaluating it. The near financial disaster of two years ago and members' initial rejections of the dues increase have made the Board more keenly aware of the responsibilities than anyone can imagine," he said.

ASRT opened its office in Albuquerque on Aug. 22, 1983. The site, which measured 20,750 square feet, was financed for $850,000 with industrial development bonds. Half the available space was rented to another organization to provide additional revenue for the Society. The Board of Directors touted the office relocation as "one of the most significant accomplishments of the Society in our history, representing a significant investment in the future stability of ASRT." By 1987 — just six years after its financial crisis and four years after its relocation to Albuquerque — the ASRT had more than $2.5 million in securities and investments.

Hardly after it had unpacked in Albuquerque, however, the Society was forced into another licensure battle with the federal government.

In 1981, when Congress passed the Radiation Health and Safety Act, it directed the U.S. Department of Health and Human Services to set minimum standards for the certification of technologists and provide a model licensure bill to the states. HHS not only ignored the Congressional order, but in July 1985 proposed that the act be repealed altogether. HHS Secretary Margaret M. Heckler asked for the repeal, stating, "Federal minimum standards in this area are cumbersome, duplicate standards developed by voluntary accrediting agencies, and have not been shown to affect radiologic safety." HHS claimed the main danger of radiation overexposure came from faulty machinery or physicians who ordered excessive x-ray exams, not from equipment operators who had never been educated as radiologic technologists.

The ASRT, estimating that nearly one-third of those performing radiographic exams in the United States still were not certified or licensed, on Aug. 14, 1985, filed a civil action suit against Heckler and the Health and Human Services department. Explaining the move, ASRT President Roland Clements, R.T.(R), said, "The secretary has failed to carry out the responsibilities and duties assigned in the Consumer-Patient Radiation Health and Safety Act of 1981. No standards have been issued and no model statute has been provided to the states. It is our opinion that the public's right to protection from radiation has thereby been neglected and disregarded."

The move by ASRT drew widespread praise, even attracting the attention of consumer advocate Ralph Nader. In an interview with the *Washington Post*, Nader criticized HHS, commenting, "This situation reveals either the bureaucratic paralysis or the lawlessness that afflicts that department on matters relating to safety. It also shows that statutory deadlines are not enough. There have to be sanctions against the bureaucrats who violated them."

Under pressure from the public and faced with a lawsuit its own attorneys believed could not be won, HHS backed down and on Oct. 11, 1985, agreed to comply with the act. It published certification and education standards in the *Federal Register* on Dec. 16 and later that month mailed copies of the standards, plus a model licensure bill, to the governors of all 50 states. The victory enhanced ASRT's growing reputation.

By this time, the ASRT found itself in a new realm. It was no longer a small family of radiologic technologists, but a large national association feeling the pressure to meet the needs of diverse groups. Other organizations representing imaging modalities such as sonogra-

phy, nuclear medicine technology and magnetic resonance imaging had formed and stood to challenge the ASRT's services and membership. Special-interest organizations devoted to radiologic science educators, department managers and administrators also emerged. The Society was concerned about adequately representing the many modalities and interests to avoid any "further fragmentation of the radiologic technology profession."

But before it could re-establish itself as the umbrella organization for all radiologic technologists, the Society first had to streamline its cumbersome organizational structure. In the early 1980s, the ASRT appointed an ad hoc committee to research the bylaws, articles of incorporation and representative structure of 30 similar medical organizations. It found the ASRT was the only one not using a delegate system. The committee recommended a complete reorganization of the Society, establishing a multidiscipline Board of Directors and a House of Delegates.

In 1982 members approved a resolution to reorganize the ASRT. The Bylaws Committee proposed the creation of specialty sections for modalities, a House of Delegates and a restructured Board of Directors. The proposal was presented at the 1983 meeting and approved in 1984. Implementation workshops began in 1985, and the first seating of the House of Delegates, the ASRT's new governing and legislative body, occurred in 1986 in San Antonio, Texas.

The ASRT House of Delegates was modeled after the representative legislatures found in the 50 states and on Capitol Hill. The country was divided into 10 regions and the membership was divided into four modalities — radiography, nuclear medicine, radiation therapy and sonography. Each region sent one delegate representing each modality to the annual meeting of the House. This system ensured that every modality and every region had equal

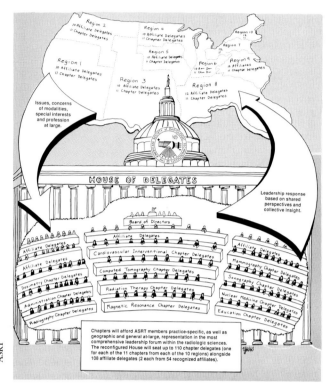

An artist's rendition of the chapters system and House of Delegates was published in a 1990 ASRT member newsletter.

representation in issues affecting the radiologic sciences. The full House also included two affiliate delegates elected from each state and city affiliate (108 total after Detroit resigned its charter). The 108 affiliate delegates plus the 40 regional modality delegates combined for a possible total of 148 House members. Delegates were encouraged to solicit opinions from their constituents, guaranteeing that all members could have a say on the future of the profession.

The Society refined the organization of its House of Delegates even further by adopting a chapter system in 1991, with full implementation in 1993. The ASRT's 20,000 members were asked to enroll in one of 11 chapters set up to provide the profession's modalities and interests better representation within the Society. The original 11 chapters were cardiovascular-interventional technology, computed tomography, dosimetry, education, magnetic

resonance, mammography, management, nuclear medicine technology, radiation therapy, radiography and sonography.

Each chapter was represented in the House by a delegate from each of the ASRT's 10 regions, replacing each region's four modality delegates. With this change, a possible total of 110 chapter delegates could serve in the House alongside the two delegates from each of the 54 affiliate societies, increasing the number of potential delegates to 218. A military chapter was added in 1995, bringing the number of chapters to 12.

The chapters system was not intended to create self-contained, autonomous units within the ASRT. Instead, it was meant to be a unifying force, linking the membership together while also recognizing its diversity. It improved the flow of information from members to leaders so the Society could provide better service.

By expanding representation, the chapters fulfilled the Society's goal of representing all technologists, educators and administrators working in all areas of medical imaging and radiation therapy. By early 1995, more than 25,000 members had chosen radiography as their primary ASRT chapter, with about 4,500 enrolled in the radiation therapy chapter, nearly 2,500 each in the mammography and computed tomography chapters, more than 2,300 in the management chapter, about 2,000 in the magnetic resonance imaging chapter, nearly 1,300 each in the education and cardiovascular-interventional technology chapters, more than 600 in the nuclear medicine chapter, 560 in the sonography chapter, close to 350 in the dosimetry chapter and 38 in the military chapter.

The reorganization of the Society and the implementation of chapters, although momentous, were just two events in a maelstrom of activity for the ASRT during the 1980s and early '90s. Also emerging during this period were an ASRT Educational Foundation, a member recruitment/retention program and the creation of National Radiologic Technology Week, an annual celebration recognizing technologists' contributions to health care. But without question, one of the biggest challenges of the era was the profession's struggle to attain majority representation on the boards of the American Registry of Radiologic Technologists and the Joint Review Committee on Education in Radiologic Technology.

The ARRT and JRCERT boards both were comprised of an equal number of ASRT-appointed technologists and ACR-appointed physicians. The possibility existed that the technologists and radiologists on the boards could vote as blocs, resulting in stalemate. At the 1982 ASRT Annual Conference, members asked the ASRT Board of Directors to seek a majority representation of technologists on both boards. They believed it was important to attain a majority on the boards so that technologists could control the future of educational programs and accreditation and certification activities.

"Technologists believed they had come into their own. They were knowledgeable and aware of what was needed in a quality education program," explained Joan Parsons, R.T.(R), who served on the Task Force on Majority Representation in 1986-87 and as ASRT president in 1989-90.

Chaired initially by Jane Van Valkenburg, R.T.(R)(N), FASRT, the Task Force on Majority Representation devised a three-part plan to secure majority representation within three years. The first step included analyzing the bylaws of the ARRT and JRCERT to find ways to achieve majority representation and collecting information on similar organizations and institutions that had achieved majority representation, such as the American Society of Medical Technologists. The second step involved contacting the ACR to solicit physi-

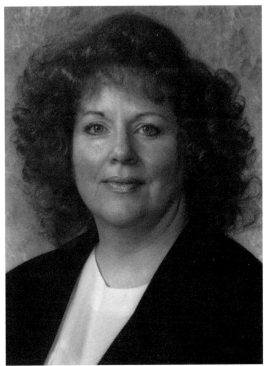

Joan Parsons served as ASRT president in 1989-90 and became executive vice president of operations in 1993.

cian support for a technologist majority on both boards. If the second step failed, technologists would advance to the third step, which involved the establishment of independent accrediting and certifying agencies.

Although this third step was viewed strictly as a last resort, technologists knew they had to be prepared to act on it. "The time has come in the history of our profession that we as technologists must determine our own destiny," announced Bill May, R.T.(R), ASRT president in 1983.

The ASRT first asked its appointees to the ARRT and JRCERT boards to present majority representation proposals at each of their meetings. The physicians on both boards, however, repeatedly defeated the proposals by stalemate. The barrage of requests created tension among board members and impeded ASRT's progress.

Phyllis Thompson, R.T.(R)(T), FASRT, an

Building a Foundation

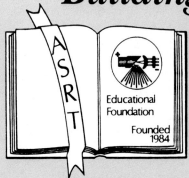

The American Society of Radiologic Technologists was founded in 1920 on a simple premise: technologist helping technologist. In the years since then, the Society has depended upon the strength of its members working in collaboration, whether fighting for state licensure or striving to elevate educational standards. No effort of the Society better exemplifies that concept than the ASRT Educational Foundation, created in 1984 to provide low-cost, quality educational materials for all radiologic technologists.

The Society benefited from charitable contributions since its beginning, but never solicited funds in an organized way. With the growing emphasis on technologist education in the early 1980s, Society leaders began talking about establishing a mechanism for corporations and individuals to make tax-deductible donations earmarked for educational programs. The Educational Foundation, established as a separate, nonprofit subsidiary of the ASRT, became that mechanism. The Foundation represented the Society's commitment to life-long learning for technologists.

The Educational Foundation held its organizational meeting June 13-14, 1984, in conjunction with the ASRT Annual Conference. Appointed to the Foundation's first Board of Directors were Tom Kraker, R.T.(R); Becky Kruse, R.T.(R); and Bill May,

R.T.(R). Kruse, who later became the Foundation's first chairman, also holds the distinction of contributing the first dollar to the Foundation's coffers.

"After the board meeting during the Annual Conference, I wanted to donate the first dollar, but all I had was a bunch of change," said Kruse. "I turned to Bill May and asked him if I could borrow a dollar, but didn't say why. He handed me the dollar and then I gave it to Ward Keller for the Foundation. Both of them wanted to make the first donation, but I beat them to the punch!"

The Foundation got off to a strong start, identifying more than 200 corporations as potential donors and also soliciting donations from hospitals, radiologists and individual technologists. By 1989, its fund balance had reached $392,289 and the Foundation was responsible for a large collection of homestudies, videotapes and seminars.

In fact, the Educational Foundation soon became the primary source of continuing education products and seminars for radiologic technologists. In 1991, however, the responsibility for developing educational materials and programs was transferred to the ASRT, leaving the Foundation free to focus exclusively on fund raising. The Foundation, thus, provides the financial support for the Society's educational efforts.

As the Foundation's focus changed, so too did the composition of its board. Today, the Educational Foundation's Board of Trustees is comprised of 10 members — seven of whom are directors of the ASRT and three of whom are members of the profession or representatives of corporations that supply goods and services to the profession.

The Foundation faced its greatest challenge with the emergence of mandatory continuing education in the early 1990s. Under pressure to fund more educational activities and ensure that quality educational programs were available to all technologists, the Foundation launched an aggressive fund-raising campaign. Contributors answered the call, and in 1992 the Foundation surpassed its $100,000 fund-raising goal by more than $50,000, thanks in large part to a $60,000 donation from Sanofi Winthrop Pharmaceuticals (now known as Nycomed). Contributions set another record high of $219,985 in 1993. The money was used to fund scholarships and produce educational courses, videotapes and homestudies — all as part of the Foundation's commitment to keeping education as affordable and accessible as possible.

At its 1993 planning meeting, the Foundation Board of Trustees set a demanding fund-raising goal: $500,000 by 1996. Helping the Foundation meet that goal was the single largest corporate gift in the Foundation's history, an $80,000 grant from Squibb Diagnostics, now known as Bracco Diagnostics. The donation was presented to the Foundation in 1993 to underwrite a series of educational videotapes. In 1994 the ASRT, as the Foundation's parent organization, contributed $100,000 in recognition of its strong financial performance throughout the year, and in 1995 Bracco again generously pledged $80,000. Also in 1995, the ASRT contributed another $100,000 to establish an endowment fund for the Educational Foundation. The endowment will create permanent investment income for the Foundation.

The Educational Foundation helped forge a link between companies affiliated with the radiologic sciences and the technologists they serve. Corporations that have shown their support for the ASRT Educational Foundation through the years include E-Z-Em Inc., Eastman Kodak, GE Medical Systems, Konica Medical Corporation, Mallinckrodt Medical Systems, Philips Medical Systems, Picker International Inc., 3M Medical Imaging, Siemens Medical Systems Inc., Varian Oncology Systems and many, many others.

Although the majority of contributions come from corporate sources, affiliate societies and hundreds of ASRT members also donate to the Foundation every year, making the Foundation truly a grassroots effort. By contributing to the ASRT Educational Foundation, technologists and corporations are investing in the future of radiologic technology.

It's as true today as it was when the Society was established in 1920: Education is the profession's foundation.

—Barbara Pongracz-Bartha

ASRT appointee to the JRCERT board in 1984, then suggested that technologists attempt to gain majority representation on the JRCERT board by "soliciting nominations from external organizations and institutions." In other words, a third organization would join the ASRT and ACR in appointing members to the JRCERT and ARRT boards.

In 1986 the ACR endorsed the Association of Educators in the Radiological Sciences, a group of educators from college-based and hospital-based programs, as an acceptable third organization. During the next year several objections arose regarding the appropriateness of the educators' association appointing technologists to the ARRT and JRCERT boards. The Utah Society of Radiologic Technologists issued a statement saying that AERS did not adequately represent its technologists. The Ohio Society, on the other

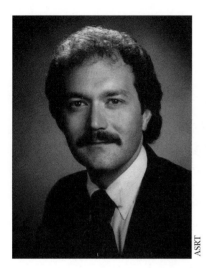 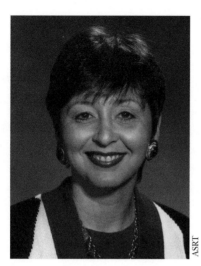 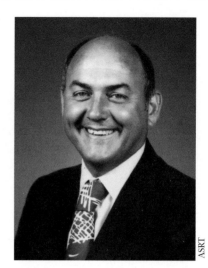

In 1991, ASRT appointees Bill May, Linda Wingfield and Roland Clements negotiated technologist majority represen-tation on the JRCERT Board of Directors.

hand, asked whether it mattered who appointed the technologists as long as they had majority representation on both boards.

In June 1988 the ASRT House of Delegates voted down AERS as an appointing organiza-tion and reassigned the Task Force on Major-ity Representation to investigate establishing a separate accreditation agency. This action sent many members into a panic; they believed the directive was tantamount to mutiny against longstanding agencies that directly affected the profession as a whole. JRCERT supporters submitted several resolu-tions to the 1990 House of Delegates asking that the task force immediately be dissolved.

Recalling the confusion surrounding the issue, Joan Parsons said, "We were presumed guilty by making the statement about inde-pendent credentialing and accreditation agencies. Even though they would have been separate entities from the Society, many peo-ple thought ASRT would control them. That was never our intent. We needed to know how to establish an independent accrediting body if that was the only way to achieve technolo-gist majority representation. We examined how it would affect ASRT and the medical imaging community."

The task force weighed several options, even asking ACR to consider appointing one less physician to obtain technologist majority representation. The ASRT also re-petitioned both the ARRT and JRCERT boards in the fall of 1990 for technologist majority representa-tion, emphasizing that ASRT was the only organization representing the "broadest spec-trum of technologist disciplines."

In March 1991 physicians on the JRCERT board again defeated the petition by stale-mate and ASRT appointees Bill May, Roland Clements, R.T.(R), FASRT, and Linda Wing-field, R.T.(R)(T), walked out of the meeting several times to protest what they later called "the radiologists' maneuvers blocking ASRT majority representation."

Recalling that dramatic meeting, May said, "We had finished our accrediting agenda and moved onto the revised bylaws, which includ-ed majority representation. The radiologists refused to vote on them. We boycotted the meeting until the radiologists agreed to vote. The radiologists called the JRCERT lawyer and said we'd abrogated our duties as board members, but we'd settled the accrediting business earlier — the JRCERT's primary responsibility."

The radiologists' actions influenced the ASRT House of Delegates decision to pass several resolutions on the issue in June 1991. The House directed a new task force to develop a plan and implementation schedule for an independent accrediting agency to present to the 1992 House of Delegates. The House also compromised on the AERS issue, approving a resolution directing the ASRT appointees to the JRCERT to pursue "two additional technologist appointments, one appointed by the ASRT and one by the AERS, creating a board of three radiologists and five technologists... and that the ASRT appointees to the ARRT continue to seek ASRT member majority representation on that board through similar avenues."

In May's opinion, "The radiologists were trying to use the AERS appointment to divide the technologists. But the physicians hadn't expected the House of Delegates to approve both an AERS and an ASRT appointee to the JRCERT board."

Technologist appointees to the ARRT Board of Trustees, however, weren't happy with the resolution. "The ARRT appointees disagreed with the last part of the resolution," said Becky Kruse, R.T.(R), a Registry board member from 1986 to 1994. "We didn't think it was right to have a specialty organization on the ARRT board, because the Registry represented all technologists and so did ASRT. AERS represented only educators. At least one of the ASRT appointees to the Registry was also a member of AERS, so already they had indirect representation on the board. We decided to continue to fight for ASRT majority representation and not compromise by introducing AERS to the Registry board."

The summer of 1991 was fairly quiet. The ASRT appointees to the JRCERT board notified the ASRT that progress was being made and asked to continue discussions.

The discussions paid off. On Sept. 14,

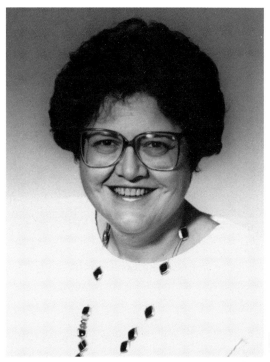

Becky Kruse has served the profession in many capacities: as ASRT president in 1984-85, as an original member of the Educational Foundation Board and as a Registry trustee from 1986 to 1994. In 1994 she was named the Society's director of continuing education.

1991, the JRCERT board approved an amendment raising the board's numbers from six to eight members by adding two additional technologists, making the balance five technologists and three physicians. One of the new technologist members would be appointed by the ASRT and the other would be named by AERS. The decision marked the end of years of negotiation and was particularly satisfying because it received unanimous approval from the JRCERT board. In a letter to the ASRT, members of the JRCERT board wrote, "This accomplishment would not have occurred without the unified effort by the members of the ASRT."

Bill May later credited the action taken by the ASRT House of Delegates in June as a deciding factor in the vote. "My opinion is

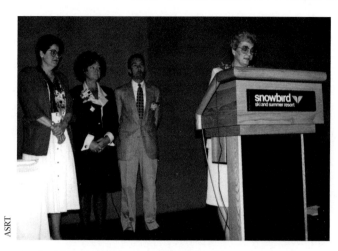

At the 1992 ASRT Annual Conference, Registry trustee Jane Van Valkenburg announced technologist majority representation on the ARRT board. Looking on are fellow trustees Becky Kruse, Belinda Phillips and Sal Martino.

that the ACR was concerned that we would have established our own accrediting organization," he said. "Going into the meeting all three of us were uncertain as to what the outcome would be. Things were pretty tense, but after about a 15-minute discussion we took the vote. We never, ever thought we would see a unanimous vote."

According to May, the ACR-appointed radiologists on the JRCERT board were concerned that if the ASRT established an independent accrediting agency, physicians would not be allowed any representation on the board of the new agency. By permitting a majority of technologists on the JRCERT board, the radiologists would be outnumbered but could maintain their input, May said.

The victory, although welcomed, was conditional. Technologists gained a majority on the JRCERT board, but ASRT and AERS would be challenged to maintain an alliance with each other.

The compromises made to obtain a technologist majority on the JRCERT board strengthened the resolve to fight for complete majority representation by technologists on the Registry Board of Trustees. That struggle

continued for another nine months. In early 1992 the ARRT bylaws were rewritten to include technologist majority representation and presented to the ARRT board at its meeting during the ASRT Annual Conference in Snowbird, Utah.

The Registry board spent Friday, June 12, strategizing and discussing the issue. On June 15, 1992, Jane Van Valkenburg, president of the board, appeared before the conference opening session to announce the unanimous passage of majority representation for technologists. ASRT would be allowed to appoint one more technologist to the Registry board, increasing the number to five, while the ACR continued to appoint four radiologists.

Van Valkenburg said the threat of ASRT establishing independent agencies if ACR didn't negotiate majority representation got ACR's attention, but wasn't the only factor in the decision. "Over the years, we built a level of trust and sincerity that I think ultimately swayed the ACR," she noted.

On July 1, 1993, Robert J. Walker, R.T.(R), became the fifth technologist on the ARRT Board of Trustees, joining fellow technologists Becky Kruse, Salvatore T. Martino, R.T.(R), Edwin J. Dice, R.T.(R)(N), and Belinda H. Phillips, R.T.(R)(T). With the implementation of the new nine-person board, changes to ARRT policies and the rules and regulations required a simple majority vote. However, election of board officers, dissolution of the ARRT, employment of the ARRT executive director, revocation of ARRT certificates, setting pass/fail scores and new ARRT exam approval required a two-thirds vote. Each board member would continue to serve a four-year term.

The successful culmination of the 10-year quest for majority representation on the JRCERT and ARRT boards meant technologists would have more influence over the future of their profession. They did not want freedom to practice their profession independent of radiologists and other physicians, but the opportunity to set their own standards. By holding a majority on both boards, technologists could influence decisions on curriculum, exam topics and accrediting criteria, as well as on one particularly contentious issue that had been needling the profession for several years — mandatory continuing education.

The seeds for mandatory continuing education were planted in the mid-'80s, when the ASRT and ARRT were trying to consolidate two different versions of a code of ethics for the profession.

"It was contradictory to have two codes of ethics since both organizations worked so closely," said Becky Kruse. "Technologists didn't know which code to follow and it threatened to split the profession." Technologist appointees to the ARRT met with ASRT Board members to meld the two codes into one document. Included in the version they finally hammered out was a statement with broad ramifications for technologists. It read, "The registered technologist continually strives to improve knowledge and skills by participating in educational and professional activities, sharing knowledge with colleagues and investigating new and innovative aspects of professional practice. One means available to improve knowledge and skill is through professional continuing education." Both boards adopted the new code of ethics and its implicit endorsement of continuing education.

The ASRT traditionally supported continuing education, but had no way of mandating it for the profession. The ARRT, however, could mandate CE as a condition for the annual renewal of technologists' registrations. The seeds were taking root.

Before deciding to mandate continuing education, however, the ARRT board wanted proof that it was effective. Board member Jane Van Valkenburg began researching con-

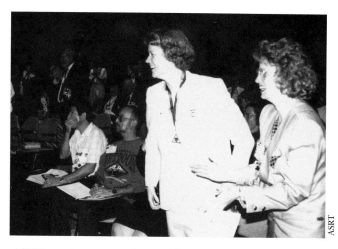

ASRT members react to the stunning announcement to appoint an additional technologist to the Registry Board. At right are Bette Schans and Kelly Thomalla.

tinuing education studies. She discovered that CE studies in the medical field had insufficient sample sizes, so she turned to studies in other technical fields such as engineering, law and education.

"Research in these areas proved that technical education directly transferred to the job," said Van Valkenburg. The ARRT accepted the results of her paper, but still faced developing a plan that would meet everyone's needs. Van Valkenburg conducted further research and wrote a proposal for implementing categorized credit.

Meanwhile, the ASRT House of Delegates in 1990 adopted a resolution submitted by the Maryland affiliate that recommended mandatory continuing education for the renewal of technologists' ARRT registrations in all disciplines. The resolution stated that mandatory continuing education would help technologists keep current with changes in their scopes of practice and professional roles, assist in attaining professional status and fully implement the code of ethics.

The ARRT developed a plan for implementing mandatory continuing education requirements, and at its February 1991 meeting the ARRT Board of Trustees voted to

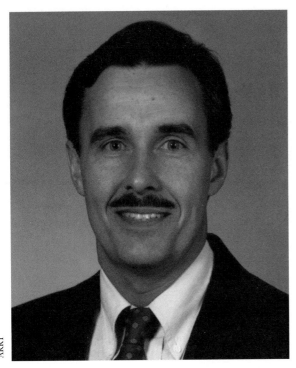

ARRT

Jerry Reid became executive director of the ARRT in 1992.

implement requirements for continuing education. The first phase of the program began Jan. 1, 1993. During this phase, technologists could accrue CE credits on a voluntary basis and receive recognition for their efforts. The second phase began Jan. 1, 1995, when technologists had to start collecting CE credits to renew the registration of their ARRT certificate. If they did not accumulate the required number of credits within a specified period they would have to retake the Registry exam or face losing their ARRT registration.

The CE requirements marked the first time in the Registry's history that renewal of a technologist's registration involved more than the submission of an application and a statement that the registrant was of good moral character. "No change at the ARRT in recent memory has had as far-reaching effects as the introduction of continuing education requirements for renewal of registration," said ARRT Executive Director Jerry Reid, Ph.D., who was promoted from director of psycho-

metric services in 1992. Reid was the first non-technologist director in the Registry's history.

Explaining the rationale behind the decision to make continuing education mandatory, Reid wrote, "Continuing education allows technologists to fulfill their responsibility to maintain competence and prevent professional obsolescence. Participation in continuing education demonstrates accountability to peers, physicians, health care facilities and the public. It also reinforces the code of ethics endorsed by the ARRT and the ASRT and recognized as the standard of conduct for radiologic technologists."

To demonstrate its commitment to continuing education as an effective way of promoting professional competence, the ASRT announced that enrollment in its Evidence of Continuing Education program, first established in 1974, would become an automatic member benefit effective Oct. 1, 1991. Under the ECE program, the Society tracks technologists' CE credits. In 1993 the ASRT also began evaluating the quality of CE activities planned by other organizations. Thus, the ASRT became one of the few organizations approved by the Registry to perform all four CE responsibilities: developing, sponsoring and evaluating continuing education activities and recording technologists' accumulated CE credits.

The requirement that technologists prove their involvement in CE activities was both hailed and reviled, easily becoming the most hotly debated issue among technologists during the early 1990s. Some technologists argued that forcing them to obtain additional education was an unfair burden, while others celebrated the opportunity to demonstrate their commitment to their profession. By the 1995 implementation date, however, debate over the issue tapered off as technologists buckled down and began collecting their CE credits. In early 1995 ASRT's membership surged to more than 44,000 — nearly doubling in just two years — as technologists turned to the Society for assistance in meeting mandatory CE requirements.

In addition to enhancing technologists' knowledge and skills, mandatory CE also was viewed by many as a route to professional status. "I believe this mandate will mean better care for our patients," ASRT President Darrell McKay, Ph.D., R.T.(R), FASRT, said in 1993. "But there is another, more subtle benefit from mandatory continuing education — it will help advance our quest to achieve professional status." McKay noted that radiologic technology could not attain professional status unless it first established uniform educational standards. Mandatory CE, he said, was the first step toward that goal.

The ultimate goal, however, may be establishing the baccalaureate degree as the entry-level standard for future technologists. The National Labor Relations Board still considers the baccalaureate degree the mark of professionalism. Through the early '90s, technologists nationwide debated entry-level requirements in the radiologic sciences. The inherent differences between hospital-based and college programs created conflicts, with inconsistent course descriptions making it difficult to transfer credits between the two types of programs.

In 1993 the ASRT House of Delegates passed a resolution making the baccalaureate mandatory for students entering radiation therapy programs beginning in 2000. A year later the House considered a resolution to make the baccalaureate the entry-level requirement for all radiologic technologists, but instead voted to investigate the issue further.

One issue resolved during the 1990s was the personnel shortage that had besieged the profession almost since its beginning. The shortage reached crisis proportions in the mid-1980s, with qualified, registered radiologic technologists in heavy demand nationwide. The shortage gave technologists' salaries a boost, even prompting some hospitals to offer sign-on bonuses or pay relocation expenses. Many radiology departments were understaffed and technologists often were expected to work overtime to compensate, contributing to high levels of stress and burnout.

In 1988, the ASRT and 17 other organizations established the Summit on Manpower to aggressively promote radiologic technology as a career. A major public relations campaign and research studies created awareness in the allied health professions and promoted radiologic technology as a career option for high school graduates. By early 1993, however, the personnel shortage had been alleviated in most areas of the country. The Summit reorganized and directed its attention to health care reform.

And the changes in the profession didn't stop there. In the fall of 1992, the American Medical Association voted to dissolve its Committee on Allied Health Education and Accreditation, the organization that accredited U.S. programs in radiologic technology. The AMA said the decision was based on "increasing professionalism in health professions, evolution of the health care team concept, the opportunity for interprofessional cooperation, a broader base for participation and leadership and financial considerations." In particular, the 1992 amendments to the Higher Education Act of 1965 specifically stated that accrediting agencies' relationships with professional organizations must "not compromise the independence of the accreditation process." If the AMA continued to sponsor CAHEA, it would violate this law.

CAHEA notified its sponsoring organizations and review committees, the largest being the JRCERT, that a new accrediting agency would have to be established by November 1993. In May 1993, however, several radiologic science organizations rejected the proposed new accrediting agency, the Council on Accreditation of Allied Health Education Programs, calling it too bureaucratic and expensive. Members of the JRCERT Board of Directors went one step further, deciding to focus their energy on establishing the JRCERT as an independent accrediting agency.

The JRCERT petitioned the U.S. Department of Education to become an independent accrediting organization in the winter of 1993. The following January, the Department of Education granted interim recognition to the JRCERT effective June 1994 through December 1995.

The Higher Education Act's preliminary rules for implementation were published in April 1994, giving the JRCERT clearer direction in pursuing permanent status as an independent accrediting agency. The JRCERT changed its policies and procedures, bylaws and board composition to comply with the Higher Education Act amendments before presenting its application for permanent status. With these changes, the JRCERT would report directly to the Department of Education, perform unannounced site visits on hospital-based, certificate and associate programs and include public representation on its board. The unannounced site visits were required for all "vocational" education programs — those below the baccalaureate level. Also, the ASRT, AERS and ACR would be allowed only to submit a slate of nominees for the JRCERT board instead of appointing board members directly.

"The requirements of the Higher Education Act have effectively changed the process of accreditation from one of professional oversight to one of regulatory compliance," said JRCERT Executive Director Marilyn Fay, M.A., R.T.(R), in 1995. "The JRCERT believes accreditation is vital to the continued integri-

ty of radiologic science educational programs and to the profession as a whole ... without accreditation there would be no degree of assurance that quality patient care would be provided, an unconscionable action considering the many dangers of using radiation to perform diagnostic examinations," noted Fay.

With its new status as an accrediting agency, the JRCERT began revising the way it surveyed educational programs. Since its formation in 1969, the JRCERT had relied on two documents to evaluate the quality of educational programs in radiologic technology: the *Essentials and Guidelines of an Accredited Educational Program for the Radiographer* and the *Essentials and Guidelines of an Accredited Educational Program for the Radiation Therapist*. The two documents defined the minimum standards for didactic, laboratory and clinical components of all educational programs for radiologic technologists.

Beginning in 1997, however, the JRCERT will bid farewell to both sets of *Essentials* and begin performing site reviews and accreditation activities under a single set of guidelines called the *Standards for an Accredited Program in Radiologic Sciences*. The *Standards* represent a dramatic shift in emphasis for programs seeking JRCERT accreditation. While the *Essentials* assessed the learning process, the *Standards* instead will measure learning outcomes. Beverly Buck, R.T.(R)(T), 1995 chairman of the JRCERT Board of Directors, said focusing on program and student outcomes is a more effective way to measure total academic effort.

According to the JRCERT, the goals of the accreditation process using the *Standards* are to protect the student and the public, provide outcomes by which a program can establish and evaluate its assessment policies and procedures, stimulate programmatic self-improvement and provide protective measures for federal funding or financial aid.

A draft of the *Standards* was released to program directors in April 1995. Work on the document began three years earlier, when the JRCERT board and staff began researching outcomes assessment and measures. They also examined the relevance of existing *Essentials* criteria and solicited comments from educators, administrators and students regarding program outcome criteria. The JRCERT hopes to finalize the *Standards* in 1996 — the latest in a long series of revolutionary educational reforms for the profession.

Although the profession of radiologic technology underwent monumental changes during the 1980s and '90s, technologists as a group remained surprisingly consistent. An ARRT survey of registered technologists conducted in 1972 and repeated in 1991 showed that the female-to-male ratio for the profession had remained steady for nearly 20 years at 75 percent female, 25 percent male. Also unchanged, despite the introduction of entire new specialities between the dates of the two surveys, was the fact that the majority of ARRT registrants continued to hold certification in radiography only. By early 1995 there were nearly 700 accredited radiography programs, 125 accredited radiation therapy programs and more than 200,000 registered radiologic technologists in the United States, making them the largest group of "allied health" professionals in the country.

Despite the many differences represented by a group that large, radiologic technologists are more alike than they are different. Their job titles may be mammographer, radiation therapist, clinical instructor or department manager, but they all are linked by a unique legacy of commitment to their profession. During the past 100 years, radiologic technologists produced vast amounts of research, developed new techniques, designed sound systems of education and established a tradition of excellence in patient care. They ended

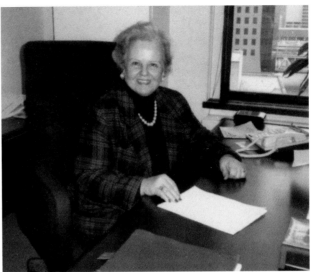

As executive director, Marilyn Fay oversaw the JRCERT's 1994 transition from a review committee to an independent accrediting agency.

their first century by embracing continuing education as proof of their commitment to professional growth.

The profession's second century will present radiologic technologists with many opportunities and challenges. On the horizon are technological innovations that can only be imagined today, plus shifts in research methods, educational paradigms, clinical practice patterns and health care delivery systems. Change will continue to be the hallmark of radiologic technology.

The profession was born when Wilhelm Conrad Roentgen carefully exposed an x-ray image of his wife's hand in 1895, but thanks to the contributions of thousands of radiologic technologists, it did not end there. As new equipment and specialties emerged, technologists adapted. As technology evolved, technologists evolved. Working in collaboration with radiologists and radiation oncologists, they helped transform the way the world diagnoses and treats disease. Radiology could not have progressed without them.

Our Destiny

If history is a journey, then radiologic technologists reached a crossroads in the early 1990s. Behind them lay the smooth trail forged by their predecessors and built upon technology, research and knowledge; ahead was an uncharted territory where virtually every aspect of the profession was undergoing rapid transformation. Unprecedented action in the arenas of education, accreditation and health care reform greeted technologists as they approached 1995, the year marking the 100th anniversary of radiology and the 75th anniversary of the ASRT. The profession's leaders urged technologists to stay informed and be proactive on issues ranging from patient-focused care and multiskilling to outcomes assessment and accreditation standards.

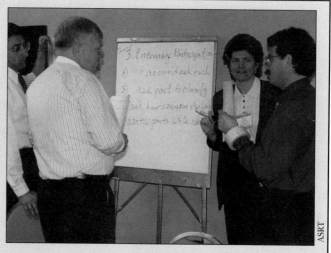

Participants in the first ASRT Educational Consensus Conference in March 1995 included radiologic science educators Michael Delvecchio, Darrell McKay and Mary Tesoriero and planning facilitator Marc Wunder.

"The most important message we need to pass on to our fellow technologists is that our future depends on the choices we make today," said ASRT President Sarah Baker, R.T.(R), FASRT, in early 1993. "We need to respond to the issues at hand and not take a 'wait-and-see' attitude. It is imperative that we take a proactive stance in the future of our profession. We must make our presence known."

Baker's words were prophetic. In November 1993 President Bill Clinton introduced a health care reform proposal in Congress designed to provide universal insurance coverage for all Americans. While Congress and the country debated the merits of the proposal, the ASRT Board of Directors discovered that Clinton's bill included a provision that could have abolished licensure laws regulating more than 600,000 U.S. health care practitioners, including radiologic technologists. The ASRT supported many aspects of the president's health reform proposal, but it could not allow reform legislation to override state licensure laws for health care professionals. It launched a letter-writing campaign among its members, urging them to voice their opposition to this provision of the president's bill. Technologists responded in full force, flooding Congress with letters and phone calls. In fact, Congress received more mail on the licensure issue than any other aspect of the health care reform bill.

Although Clinton's proposal ultimately failed, technologists' efforts caught the attention of Sen. Bob Graham, D-Fla., and Sen. James Jeffords, R-Vt., who wrote an amendment to strike from all future health care reform legislation "any provision which pre-empts or overrides the traditional authority of the states to regulate health care professionals." Radiologic technologists had again demonstrated the power of their united efforts.

But even without a mandate from Congress, the health care industry began reorganizing itself. As hospitals merged, shifted to managed care or redesigned work flow, many radiology departments saw their staffs and budgets shrink. In some institutions, radiologic technologists were asked to become cross-trained and take on additional responsibilities outside the radiology department.

Engulfed by these sweeping changes, the profession had to re-evaluate how it prepared technologists to enter clinical practice. In March 1995 the ASRT brought more than 60 radiologic science educators together for a first-of-its-kind national Educational Consensus Conference. Their findings called for dramatic changes in educational methods and clinical practice to enable the profession to reach new heights in diagnosis, service and treatment. Participants suggested that the profession implement a career ladder for technologists, with the associate degree as the educational standard for entry-level professionals and the baccalaureate degree as the standard for multicompetent professionals. They also recommended that the radiography curriculum be expanded to include a stronger foundation in general education and to teach technologists the critical-thinking, decision-making and scientific inquiry skills they will need to survive in a changing health care environment. The first conference was successful in identifying the issues facing the profession; the ASRT planned to sponsor a second Educational Consensus Conference in 1996 to determine a course of action.

As radiologic technologists enter their second century as a profession, the challenge is not just to progress, but to prosper. While no one can predict with any certainty what the future holds for radiologic technology, it is certain the ASRT will guide the way. Membership soared to more than 44,000 in 1995, with the Society representing one out of every five registered radiologic technologists in the United States. Its members are the Society's strength. Since its formation, the ASRT has attracted the profession's thinkers and visionaries — those who write, teach and organize. Their clarity of vision will continue to define the evolving profession of radiologic technology.

In 1981 ASRT Chief Executive Officer Ward Keller described the ASRT's commitment to the future. "Progress has been the vital watchword for ASRT," he said. "Status quo has never been satisfactory, nor will it ever be. ASRT is committed to continual self-examination and readjustment. As your personal and professional needs change and develop, we are obligated to help you fulfill them. As the profession of radiologic technology grows, we are bound to grow with it. It is through progress that we serve you better and more effectively."

—*Barbara Pongracz-Bartha*

Index

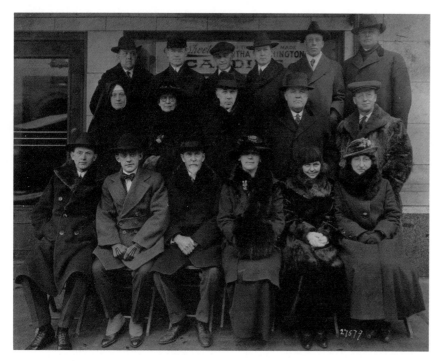

The American Society of Radiographers — as the technologists' organization was known at the time — held its 1931 annual meeting in St. Paul, Minn. President Emma Grierson (middle row, second from left) and founder Ed Jerman (bottom row, third from left) joined fellow members for this group photo.

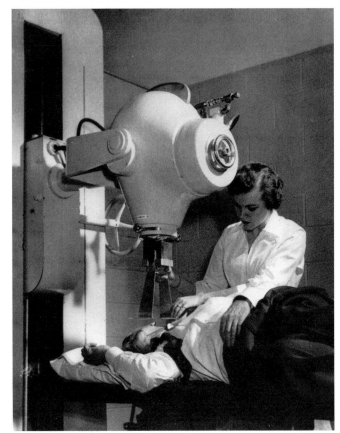

Cobalt therapy, circa 1950

An application form for ASXT membership, circa 1940.

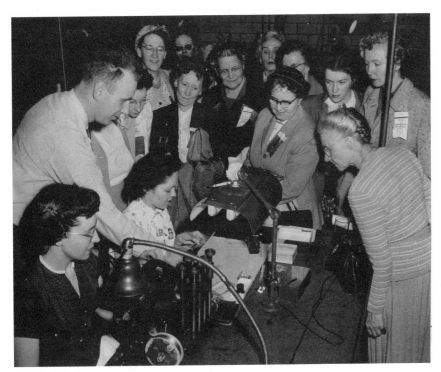

Technologists toured the General Electric plant in Milwaukee during the 1952 ASXT Annual Conference and observed the delicate job of assembling x-ray tubes.

References

Introduction

pages 1-3: Information on Wilhelm Conrad Roentgen is from *Wilhelm Conrad Roentgen and The Early History of the Roentgen Rays* by Otto Glasser (Charles C Thomas Publisher, Springfield, Ill., 1934).

Chapter 1 • Birth of a Science

pages 4-6: Ed Jerman began collecting articles from the Journal of the American Medical Association as soon as Roentgen announced his discovery. All quotations from JAMA are from Jerman's collection. These items later were published by the Victor X-Ray Corporation in its newsletter, *The Victor News.*

page 4: **"a revolting indecency..."** Quoted in *The Trail of the Invisible Light* by E.R.N. Grigg (Charles C Thomas Publisher, Springfield, Ill., 1964), p. 33.

pages 4-6: Information on the public's reaction to the x-ray is described in *Radiology, An Illustrated History*, by Ronald L. Eisenberg (Mosby Year Book Inc., St. Louis, 1992), pp. 58-59.

page 6: **"Many men attracted by the unknown..."** Wolfram Fuchs is quoted by Eisenberg, p. 58.

page 7: Walter J. Dodd's working conditions were chronicled by Eisenberg, p. 68.

page 8: **"the only valid criticism..."** Carman is quoted by Eisenberg, p. 61.

page 8: **"a heritage still remains..."** Murphy is quoted by Eisenberg, p. 60.

pages 9-10: Early safety precautions regarding the use of the x-ray are discussed by Eisenberg, pp. 158-170.

page 9: **"all those who are employed..."** Eisenberg, p. 160.

pages 10-12: Additional information on Heber Robarts and the Roentgen Society is found in Eisenberg, p. 564, and Grigg, pp. 189-205.

page 12: **"engulfed with electrotherapists..."** Grigg, p. 187.

page 12: **"undesirable elements..."** Grigg, p. 190.

page 13: **"by the time a half-dozen pictures..."** F.S. O'Hara, "Looking Backward." *Radiography and Clinical Photography.* 1932, Vol. 8, pp. 3-9.

page 14: **"Away with your stethoscope..."** From an editorial titled "Roentgen's Rays," appearing in the March 1896 issue of the *New Orleans Medical and Surgical Journal*, p. 535.

page 14: DeLaup's comments are from the Transactions of the Louisiana State Medical Society, 1899, p. 72.

page 14: **"every instrument of precision..."** From Leon J. Menville's article titled "An Obituary of Amedee Granger, M.D.," appearing in the January 1940 issue of *Radiology*, pp. 108-109. Other descriptions of equipment acquisitions and department renovations are from the 1896, 1899, 1905, 1906 and 1908 annual reports from Charity Hospital of New Orleans.

page 14: **"The increasing importance..."** Charity Hospital of New Orleans Annual Report, 1908, pp. 41-42.

page 15: The loss of 50 milligrams of radium was described in the *New Orleans Morning Tribune*, May 19, 1931, p. 1.

Chapter 2 • Enter the Specialists

page 16: **"medical radiography was a piebald proceeding..."** Percy Brown is quoted by Eisenberg, p. 58.

pages 16-18: For further information on the ARRS, Percy Brown and Russell Carman, see Eisenberg, pp. 58-59.

page 19: **"much like that of a group..."** James Case is quoted by Eisenberg, pp. 579-580.

page 19: **"the vicious tendency..."** Eisenberg, p. 580.

page 21: Information on Charles Leonard is included in Eisenberg, pp. 168-169.

pages 22-23: Information regarding the founding of the RSNA and ACR and the comments of Arthur Wright Erskine and Albert Soiland can be found in Grigg, pp. 568-569.

page 23: The dilemma of exhibition space is detailed in Eisenberg, pp. 571-572.

page 24: **"The evolution and progress..."** Eisenberg, p. 60.

pages 24-25: Information on Marie Curie is from Eisenberg, pp. 43-50, and from *Marie Curie — A Life,* by Francoise Giroud, translated by Lydia David (Holmes & Meier, 1986).

Chapter 3 • The Technician's Evangelist

pages 26-35: Information on the Jerman family and Ed Jerman's early life and career comes from an unpublished manuscript by Elmer Jerman titled "Memoirs of Ed C. Jerman" and an unpublished history titled *The Ups and Downs of An X-Ray Man's Life* by Ed C. Jerman. Both are held in the ASRT archives in Albuquerque, N.M.

Chapter 4 • A Society of Technicians

pages 38-40: Quotes about the AART originate from the minutes of the Society's first organizational meeting, minutes from the first annual meeting and *A History of the ASXT* by Margaret Hoing (Bruce Publishing Co., St. Paul, Minn., 1952).

page 41: **"commercially competitive..."** Grigg, p. 623.

pages 42-43 and 46-47: All quotations by Alfred Greene are from his *History of the Registry* and his article titled "The American Registry of X-Ray Technicians: Twenty-two Years of Achievement," in the November 1945 issue of *The X-Ray Technician*.

pages 44-45: Information on Edward Gunson is from personal interviews conducted during September 1994.

page 45: Information on Sister Mary Beatrice's Registry exam is from "First Registry Examination Discovered," *Radiologic Technology*, 1972, Vol. 42, pp. 218-219.

page 48: Information about the Society's journal is from the minutes of the 1929 AART annual meeting.

pages 49-50: Information about nuns in radiologic technology is from *Pioneer Healers: The History of Women Religious in American Healthcare* by Sister Ursula Stepsis and Sister Delores Liptak (Crossroad Publishing Co., New York, N.Y., 1989) and "Historical Considerations of the Department of Radiology of St. Mary's Infirmary, St. Louis, Mo.," a thesis written by Sister Mary Hugh Boente, St. Louis University, 1943. Quotes from Sister Agnes Therese Duffy, Sister Stella Louise Slomka, Sister Marylu Stueber and Sister Maria Elena are from personal interviews conducted during the spring of 1995.

Chapter 5 • Setting the Standards

Much of the background information for this chapter was derived from Alfred Greene's *History of the Registry*.

page 55: For more information about General Electric's patent on the Coolidge tube, see "The Life of Ed C. Jerman: A Historical Perspective," by Richard Terrass in the May/June 1995 issue of *Radiologic Technology*, pp. 291-298.

page 58: The comments by Sister Mary Beatrice Merrigan and Edward H. Skinner about Ed Jerman are from a speech by Sister Mary Beatrice presented before the 16th annual meeting of the Missouri Society of X-Ray Technicians, April 3, 1948.

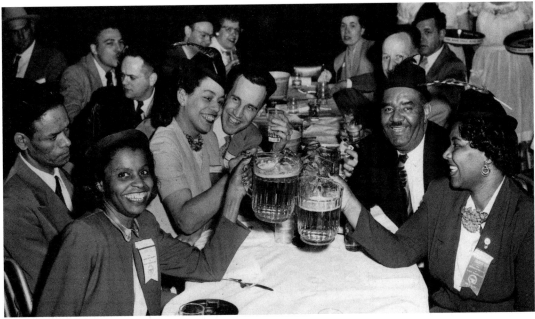

The 1952 ASXT Annual Conference, in Milwaukee, featured a German "Oktoberfest" party.

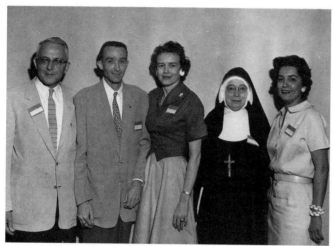

ASXT officers for 1958-59 were, from left to right, Ralph J. Bannister, president; Meredith G. Lewis, president-elect; Marjorie Tolan, first vice president; Sister Mary Beatrice Merrigan, second vice president; and Laura Seniors, secretary-treasurer.

page 61: **"Professor Ed C. Jerman..."** From an article titled "The Technician's Legacy" by Margaret Hoing, September 1948 *X-Ray Technician*, pp. 69-79.

page 61: **"Far beyond the feeling of gratitude..."** From *A History of the ASXT, 1920-1950*, by Margaret Hoing. Bruce Publishing Company, St. Paul, Minn., 1952, p. 11.

page 61: **"My mind travels along memory's trail..."** From Thomas Lough's introduction to *A History of the ASXT, 1920-1950*. Bruce Publishing Company, St. Paul, Minn., p. 9.

page 62: The resolution about trade unions is from the minutes of the 1929 AART annual meeting.

pages 64-65: For more information on the radiographer's role in mass chest x-ray surveys during the 1940s and '50s, see "A Mass X-Ray Survey from a Photofluorographic Operator's Point of View" by James H. Hennessey, R.T., in the March 1952 issue of *The X-Ray Technician* (pp. 329-337) and "Largest X-Ray Survey" in the January 1951 issue of *The X-Ray Technician* (p. 212). Tuberculosis mortality figures were obtained from Mark Caldwell's *The Last Crusade: The War on Consumption, 1862-1954*; (Macmillan Publishing Co., New York, 1988) p. 247. Also see *The Forgotten Plague: How the Battle Against Tuberculosis Was Won — And Lost*, by Frank Ryan (Little, Brown and Company, Boston, Mass., 1992).

Chapter 6 • The War Years

page 66: For further information about the U.S. medical forces in World War II, see *Radiology in WWII* by Leonard Heaton (Office of the Surgeon General, U.S. Army Medical Department, Washington, D.C., 1966).

page 66: For further information about Lt. Colonel de Lorimer, see Heaton, pp. 24-28.

page 68: **"de Lorimer's 8-week wonders..."** Heaton, p. 28.

page 68: **"because of patriotic reasons..."** *The X-Ray Technician*, March 1941, p. 199.

page 68: Information about rumored training programs to replace civilian technologists with those trained in the military can be found in *The X-Ray Technician*, March 1941, p. 199, and March 1942, pp. 217-18.

page 68: The salaries of military x-ray technicians and junior laboratory helpers is detailed in *The X-Ray Technician*, July 1942, p. 37.

page 68: **"Careful investigation..."** *The X-Ray Technician*, May 1944, p. 256.

page 69: Information on 90-day military x-ray training programs is from *Radiologic Technology*, November 1986, pp. 123-133.

page 69: Information about technologists' struggle for recognition by the AMA can be found in "The Registry Comes of Age," a series of articles by Alfred B. Greene appearing in *The X-Ray Technician* from January through July 1944.

page 70: **"The present world crisis..."** *The X-Ray Technician*, November 1942, p. 126.

page 70: Additional information on technologist "raids" can be found in *The X-Ray Technician*, November 1942, p. 126.

page 70: **"not all these raids..."** *The X-Ray Technician*, November 1942, p. 126.

page 70: **"it falls to the women..."** *The X-Ray Technician*, November 1942, p. 130.

page 70-71: Background information for the expectations of men and women technologists came from *The X-Ray Technician*, May 1941, pp. 207 and 250, and September 1943, p. 60.

page 72: **"impede or interfere..."** *The X-Ray Technician*, January 1943, p. 174.

page 73: Further information on the AMA approval of x-ray schools and the evolution of educational standards can be found in *The X-Ray Technician*, September 1941, pp. 79-80.

page 73: Information about the establishment of the Canadian Registry is found in *The X-Ray Technician*, May 1944, p. 258, as part of "The Registry Comes of Age" series by Alfred B. Greene.

pages 74-76: The quotes and background research of the radiologic scenarios in the European and Pacific theaters during World War II are from Heaton, pp. 327-380 and pp. 519-608.

page 76: **"use sparingly and with great care…"** *The X-Ray Technician*, March 1943, p. 209.

page 76: Additional information on Arthur W. Fuchs is found in *Radiologic Technology*, January/February 1987; information on the betatron is found in Grigg, pp. 340-48.

page 76: **"though we did make one six-hour…"** *The X-Ray Technician*, July 1945, pp. 235-36.

page 77: **"Looking to the future…"** *The X-Ray Technician*, July 1943, p. 29.

page 77-78: **"devil-dancer"** and other related quotes are detailed in *The X-Ray Technician*, July 1943, p. 28-29.

page 78: Information about Rose Marie Pegues and the history of African-Americans in radiologic technology is courtesy of Alan Oestreich, Children's Hospital Medical Center, Cincinnati, Ohio.

page 79: Quotes from Theodore Ott are from personal interviews conducted during the fall of 1994 and spring of 1995.

Chapter 7 • The Emergence of Excellence

page 80: "Men, and especially women…" From an article titled "From G.I. to R.T." by F.F. Schweitzer in *The X-Ray Technician*, March 1947, pp. 223-225.

page 82: Information on changes in the Registry exam format was provided by Jerry Reid during personal interviews.

page 82-83: **"Sad to say…"** From an editorial titled "A Prevalent Fallacy" in *The X-Ray Technician*, January 1942, pp. 159-160.

pages 83-84: X-ray technicians' efforts in civil defense are chronicled in the following articles, all from *The X-Ray Technician*: "The X-Ray Technician and the Atomic Age," by Ellis J. Wick, March 1950, pp. 284-287; "President's Message," by John Cahoon, November 1950, p. 173; "Civil Defense and You," by Richard Olden, July 1951, pp. 37-38; "The X-Ray Technician and the Atomic Bomb," by Harold J. Peggs, July 1951, pp. 10-12; "Report of Special Committee on Civil Defense,"

September 1951, pp. 143-144; "Civil Defense — Let's Face It," by Dewey Blackstone, January 1952, pp. 283-284; and "Medical Aspects of an Atomic Explosion," by Everett Pirkey, July 1952, pp. 8-9.

page 85: Keichline's and Clarke's comments on the age requirement are from an article titled "Registry Board Quiz Session" in *The X-Ray Technician*, November 1947, pp. 130-137.

page 85: Discussion of additional credentials can be found in an article titled "ARXT Panel Discussion" in *The X-Ray Technician*, September 1950, pp. 84-86.

page 87: Richard Olden's comments about the shortage of x-ray technicians are from his President's Message in the November 1953 issue of *The X-Ray Technician*, pp. 186-187.

page 87: More information about the "Philadelphia Plan" can be found in two articles from *The X-Ray Technician*: "First Class Graduates Under Philadelphia Plan," July 1953, pp. 47-49; and "Second Class Graduated by Philadelphia Plan," September 1954, pp. 113-114.

page 87: **"There is little uniformity…"** From "The Future Belongs to You," by Richard Olden, *The X-Ray Technician*, September 1952, pp. 112-114.

pages 87-88: For more information about the minimum curricula, see "A Basic Curriculum in X-Ray Technology," *The X-Ray Technician*, November 1952, pp. 218-219.

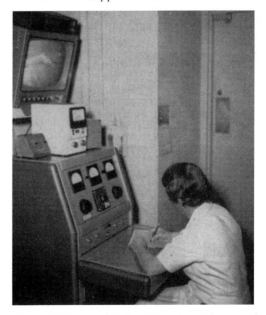

Circa 1961 – A radiation therapist at the controls of a Van de Graaf machine.

page 88: Allen's comments are from "The Professional Status of the X-Ray Technician," *The X-Ray Technician*, September 1948, pp. 109-110.

pages 89-90: Quotes from Genevieve Eilert are from personal interviews.

page 91: A full transcript of the ASXT panel discussion on state licensure is included in an article titled "State Licensure," *The X-Ray Technician*, March 1949, pp. 259-266.

page 91: **"If your national society…"** From an article by Mac Cahal titled "Did You Call, Doctor?" in *The X-Ray Technician*, January 1947, pp. 155-157.

page 91: The ASXT resolution opposing licensure was printed in the September 1948 issue of *The X-Ray Technician*, p. 112.

page 92: Information on film processing is from Eisenberg, pp. 93-94.

page 92: The quote about technicians' professionalism is from "The Professional Status of the X-Ray Technician," *The X-Ray Technician*, September 1948, pp. 109-110.

pages 93-94: Information on ASXT Annual Conferences was compiled from reports in *The X-Ray Technician*. Melvin Aspray's comments are from the July 1949 issue; John Cahoon's are from the September 1950 issue. Information on the 1954 meeting in Miami is from the January 1954 issue, page 294. Jack Cullinan's comments are from personal communications.

Chapter 8 • A New Generation of Giants

Quotations in this chapter from Frances Apple, Bill Conklin, Virginia Milligan, Ruth Jaffke, Royce Osborn, Ted Ott, Jack Cullinan and Angie Cullinan are from personal interviews conducted during the fall and winter of 1994.

pages 94, 96: Clark Warren's comments about the creation of the Fellow category are from "Accomplishments and Opportunities," *The X-Ray Technician*, September 1956, pp. 109-115.

pages 99-100, 101: The comments by Cynthia Easterling about John Cahoon are from her 1978 Cahoon Memorial Lecture titled "What Price Professionalism?"

page 102: **"The greatest that I have ever…"** Margaret Hoing, *The X-Ray Technician*, March 1946, p. 417.

page 105: **"Possessed a drive, a dedication…"** Jean Widger, "Is Excellence Still Respectable?" *Radiologic Technology*, January 1970, pp. 219-231

Chapter 9 • Technician Becomes Technologist

pages 112-113: **"The simple triad…"** John Cahoon, "New Horizons in the Technical and Educational Systems of Radiologic Technology." *Radiologic Technology*, November 1970, pp. 83-90.

page 113: Information on the report by the Surgeon General's National Advisory Committee on Radiation is from a speech made by Laurence Robbins at the 1966 ASRT Annual Conference. Robbins' speech was printed in *Radiologic Technology*, September 1966, pp. 82-83.

page 113: Recommendations from the 1966 National Conference on X-Ray Technician Training were reported in *Radiologic Technology*, November 1966, pp. 175-179.

page 113: **"Licensure of radiologic technologists…"** *Radiologic Technology*, January 1965, pp. 336-337.

pages 114-116: Background information on radiologic technologists who served in the Vietnam War was obtained from three articles in *Radiologic Technology*: "Technicians for South Vietnam," July 1964, pp. 91-92; "Technicians for Vietnam," September 1964, p. 191; and Juris Patrylak's "X-Ray Technology Aboard the Hospital Ship U.S.S. Sanctuary," January 1972, pp. 278-281. Additional information is from "The Legacy of the White Lily Fleet," by Cdr. Paul N. Grinkevich, which appeared in the April 1987 issue of *The Retired Officer*, pp. 27-31; and *The American Experience in Vietnam* by Clark Dougan and Stephen Weiss (W.W. Norton & Company, New York, N.Y., 1988). All quotes and reminiscences of Juris Patrylak, R.T., are based on personal interviews conducted in April 1995.

page 116-117: **"The Registry figures will attest…"** Patricia J. O'Reilly, "President's Message." *Radiologic Technology*, March 1964, p. 407.

pages 117-118: Information on Sen. Bartlett's hearings is from Warren H. Donnelly's article titled "Bushwhacking, Licensure and Senator Bartlett." *Radiologic Technology*, November 1971, pp. 248-258.

page 117: **"We believe that federal minimum standards…"** Leslie Wilson, "Statement of the American Society of Radiologic Technologists to the Senate Committee on Commerce." *Radiologic Technology*, July 1968, pp. 33-37.

pages 118-119: **"This Society will fight…"** Royce Osborn, "Your ASRT President Comments." *ASRT Scanner*, June 1970, p. 2.

page 119: More information on the 1978 revision of the *Essentials* may be found in "Status of the Essentials" by Virginia Milligan, *Radiologic Technology*, May 1978, pp. 782-784; and "Essentials Hearing a Success," *ASRT Scanner*, April 1978, p. 1. Richard Bower's quote is from his "President's Message" in *Radiologic Technology*, Nov. 1978, pp. 316-317.

page 120: **"It is my earnest hope…"** Speech by Jennings Randolph reprinted in *Radiologic Technology*, November 1977, pp. 361-387.

page 120: Salary information for radiologic technologists is from "Survey Report of Pay, Benefits and Working Conditions," *Radiologic Technology*, July 1967, pp. 51-64. Information comparing salaries of technologists and nurses is from "Tell It Like It Is," *ASRT Scanner*, December 1972, p. 2.

page 120: The growth of unions in hospitals was reported in Richard Laner's article titled "Employer-Employee Relations: Unions and Hospitals." *Radiologic Technology*, July 1974, pp. 10-14.

page 121: **"Unions view the R.T.…"** From *ASRT Scanner*, "Legislation to Affect Radiologic Technologists," February 1972, pp. 1-4.

page 121: **"To call the ASRT a union…"** Robert Best, "R.T.s are Different." *ASRT Scanner*, October 1972, p. 2.

pages 121-122: The discrepancy between salaries of male and female technologists was reported in "Profile of Members of the ASRT Including Salary Comparisons," *Radiologic Technology*, July 1972, pp. 26-31.

page 122: Bill Conklin's comments are from his article titled "The Salary Dilemma of Radiologic Technologists in South Carolina," *ASRT Scanner*, October 1972, p. 2.

page 123: The ACR position statement recognizing radiologic technologists as professionals was printed in the October 1980 *ASRT Presidential Newsletter*, p. 1.

pages 123-124: Daniel Donohue's House testimony was printed in the August 1979 issue of *ASRT Scanner*, p. 1.

page 124: **"As the supervisors…"** James Steele's Senate testimony was reported in "Special Report on Senate Bill 667," *Radiologic Technology*, November 1974, pp. 152-188.

page 124: Jean Widger's comments about licensure are from her article titled "Limited Licensure and Public Protection," *Radiologic Technology*, May 1978, pp. 779-782.

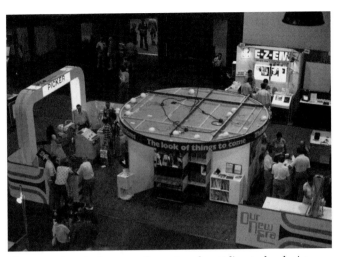

Eager to view the latest equipment and supplies, technologists crowded the exhibit hall at the 1978 ASRT Annual Conference in Anaheim, Calif.

page 124: **"We remain firm in our opinion…"** From "Statement of Donohue Before Senate Subcommittee," *Radiologic Technology*, July 1980, pp. 79-81.

pages 124-125: Comments by Ward Keller about the passage of the Radiation Health and Safety Act are from personal interviews.

pages 125-127: More information about radiologic technologists who served aboard the S.S. Hope can be found in the following articles, all from *Radiologic Technology:* "A Technologist's Year on the Ship Hope," March 1966, pp. 337-346; "Technologist on Fifth Hope Trip," July 1968, pp. 90-91; "S.S. Hope X-Ray Department Serves Needs of Needy," March 1971, pp. 430-431.

Chapter 10 • The Healing Rays

page 128: For more information on Emil Grubbé's experiments, see Paul C. Hodge's *The Life and Times of Emil H. Grubbé* (University of Chicago Press, Chicago, Ill., 1964), pp. 5-30.

page 128: **"any physical agent…"** Gilman quoted in *The Rays: A History of Radiology in the United States and Canada*, by Ruth and Edward Brecher (Williams and Wilkins, Baltimore, Md., 1969), p. 94.

page 128: **"For the first time in history…"** Grubbé quoted by Brecher and Brecher, p. 95.

page 130: Heber Robarts quoted by Brecher and Brecher, p. 146.

page 130-131: Information about tube voltages is from "The Early History of Radiotherapy" by Manuel Lederman, *International Journal of*

Radiation Oncology, Biology and Physics, May 1981, pp. 639-648.

page 130: Details about radium supply and price in 1903 are from *Principles of Radiation Therapy* by Thomas J. Deeley (Butterworth & Co. Ltd., London, 1976), pp. 12-19; and "The American Radium Society: Its Diamond Jubilee," by J.A. del Regato, *American Journal of Clinical Oncology*, Vol. 14, 1991, pp. 93-100.

page 131: For more information on Albert Soiland, see "Albert Soiland and the Early Development of Therapeutic Radiology in the United States" by J.A. del Regato, *International Journal of Radiation Oncology, Biology and Physics*, February 1983, pp. 243-253.

page 131: The supervoltage unit at St. Bartholomew's is described in "Development of the Technology of Radiation Therapy" by John S. Laughlin, *RadioGraphics*, November 1989, pp. 1245-1266.

page 131: Development of the cyclotron is described by Brecher and Brecher, pp. 364-370.

page 133: **"where we as technicians..."** Donalee L. Tabern, "Diagnostic Procedures with Radioisotopes." *The X-Ray Technician*, July 1955, pp. 32-38.

pages 133-134: A discussion of the evolution of cobalt 60 therapy may be found in John S. Laughlin's "Development of the Technology of Radiation Therapy," *RadioGraphics*, November 1989, pp. 1245-1266.

pages 133-134: For a complete description of Leonard Grimmett's development of the first cobalt 60 unit, see Grigg, pp. 301-303.

page 134: Statistics on supervoltage units during 1968 are from Brecher and Brecher, p. 354.

page 135: **"No longer can a general staff technologist..."** Colleen Pearce and John Webster, "Radiation Therapy Technology: Problems and Progress." *Radiologic Technology*, July 1971, pp. 1-6.

page 135: **"Radiation therapy as a specialty..."** Franz Buschke, "Radiation Therapy: The Past, the Present, the Future." *American Journal of Roentgenology*, February 1970, pp. 236-246.

page 135: Quotes from Norbert Black were obtained in personal interviews conducted in June 1995.

page 136: **"The Registry, with our help..."** Patricia O'Reilly, "President's Message." *The X-Ray Technician*, September 1963, p. 96.

pages 137: Statistics on the number of educational programs during 1975 are from "JRC Profile of Education in Radiologic Technology." *Radiologic Technology*, January 1976, pp. 263-265.

page 138: The 1976 revision of the *Essentials of an Accredited Educational Program for the Radiation Therapy Technologist* was printed in the July 1977 issue of *Radiologic Technology*, pp. 21-26.

page 138: **"The 12-month program..."** Jules Rominger and Diana Browning, "Radiation Therapy Technology." *Radiologic Technology*, May 1979, pp. 720-721.

page 138: **"In 1977, a 12-month program..."** Arlene Caughron, "Radiation Therapy Revisited." *Radiologic Technology*, November 1979, pp. 344-346.

page 140: **"The consensus was..."** Beverly Buck, "President's Corner." *ASRT Scanner*, February 1989, pp. 1-2.

page 140: The Department of Labor's definition of a "professional" is from *Educating Personnel for the Allied Health Professions and Services* by E.J. McTernan and R.O. Hawkins Jr. (Mosby Year Book, St. Louis, Mo., 1972), pp. 82-83.

page 140: Statistics on educational levels are from "Entry-Level Standards for Radiation Therapists," *Radiation Therapist*, February 1993, pp. 30-41.

page 141: For more information on educational standards in other countries, see "Where In the World Are We?" by Beverly Buck, *Radiation Therapist*, January 1992, pp. 267-268.

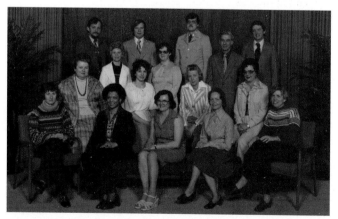

Attending a 1978 educators' seminar sponsored by Eastman Kodak were (bottom row, left to right) Jacqueline Walker, Barbara Wilson, Angie Cullinan, Frances Olson, Linda Myers; (second row, left to right) Marilyn Fay, Teresa Tucci, Florajane Holohan, Addie Haverfield; (third row, left to right) Ann Thompson, Geraldine Ruiz, Robert Dacker; (top row, left to right) William Murdoch, Randy Griswold, Jack Olley, Robert Smith.

page 141: For more information on the number of baccalaureate degree programs, see "Opinions on Baccalaureate Degrees for Radiation Therapists" by Stephanie Eatmon, J. Slater and William Preston, *Radiologic Technology,* January 1991, pp. 210-214.

page 141: Statistics on the number of certified radiation therapists is from "ARRT History Lesson" by Jerry Reid, *Radiologic Technology,* May 1995, pp. 334-336.

page 142: Salary information is from National Survey of Hospital and Medical School Salaries, University of Texas Medical Branch at Galveston, 1994.

page 142: Results of the 1993 survey of female radiation therapists is reported in "Problems Encountered in the Workplace by Female Therapists" by Judith M. Schneider, *Radiation Therapist,* October 1993, pp. 93-100.

page 142: For more information about the development of multileaf collimators, see "Optimization of Radiation Therapy and the Development of Multileaf Collimation" by Anders Brahme, *International Journal of Radiation Oncology, Biology and Physics,* Vol. 25, 1993, pp. 373-375.

page 143: Statistics on cancer cure rates are from *Cancer Facts and Figures,* published by the American Cancer Society, Atlanta, Ga., 1994.

page 143: Donna Dunn's 1979 survey was reported in her article titled "Work Values and Career Preferences of Radiation Therapy Technologists," *Radiologic Technology,* Vol. 56, 1985, pp. 326-331.

page 143: **"It's incredible how much..."** Donna Dunn, "A Look at the Radiation Therapists of Yesterday, Today and Tomorrow," *Radiation Therapist,* Fall 1994, pp. 117-118.

Chapter 11 • *Multiple Identities*
Quotations in this chapter from Laverne Gurley, Jane Van Valkenburg, Hal Magida, Louise Broadley, Joan Baker, Bill Faulkner and Carolyn Kaut Wilson are from personal interviews conducted during the fall and winter of 1994 and spring of 1995.

pages 146, 150: Information on the AURT and AERS is from Greg Spicer, "The Association of Educators in the Radiologic Sciences — A Short History," 1989, unpublished.

page 146: **"While in-service education..."** Laverne Gurley, "Inservice Education in Departments of Radiology," *Radiologic Technology,* Vol. 40, 1969, pp. 371-373.

page 147: Information on the first AHRA members is from Louise Broadley, "Fifteen Years of Growth and Progress," *Radiology Management,* Spring 1989, p. 20.

page 148: **"The early officers..."** Joan Baker, *History of Sonography.* (Smithsonian Institution, Washington, D.C., 1994), p. 22.

page 148: The letter to George Taplin is described in "A Glimpse Into the Past," *Journal of Nuclear Medicine Technology,* Vol. 13, 1985, pp. 110-112.

Chapter 12 • *New Beginnings*
Unless otherwise noted, all quotes from Joan Parsons, Becky Kruse, Bill May and Jane Van Valkenburg were obtained during personal interviews conducted in May 1995.

pages 154, 156-157: Information on the Society's financial crisis can be found in "Annual Report of the Executive Director," *Radiologic Technology,* November/December 1981, pp. 261-263; and in April 1981 through September 1981 issues of the *ASRT Scanner.*

pages 154, 156: **"We are now at the point ..."** Ward Keller, "Annual Report of the Executive Director," *Radiologic Technology,* November/December 1981, p. 261.

page 156: Information on the final vote for the dues increase is found in "Salt Lake Meeting: Members Choose Progress," *ASRT Scanner,* August/September 1981, pp. 1-2.

pages 156-158, 161-162: Information on the ASRT relocation including dollar amounts and industrial development bonds was found in the *President's Newsletter,* March 1983, pp. 1-5.

page 158: **"would not be appreciable ..."** From the *President's Newsletter,* March 1983, p. 1.

page 159: **"I am here to embark..."** From a speech delivered by David Kessler at the 1993 RSNA meeting.

page 159: Estimated number of ACR-accredited mammography sites is from the *Federal Register,* Vol. 58, No. 243, p. 67559.

page 159: **"The ACR is not a regulatory body..."** Marie Zinninger quoted in August 1994 *RS Wavelength,* p. 13.

page 159: Breast cancer statistics from American Cancer Society and Bureau of Vital Statistics.

page 160: **"If I had waited until next year..."** Marilyn Lloyd quoted in August/September 1991 *RS Wavelength,* p. 2.

page 160: Statistics on lung cancer are from *Cancer Facts and Figures 1994* (American Cancer Society, Atlanta, Ga.), 1994.

page 161: **"There were always those institutions..."** Marie Zinninger quoted in August 1994 *RS Wavelength*, pp. 12-13.

pages 161-162: **"The dues increase..."** James Mom, *President's Newsletter*, March 1983, p. 4.

page 162: **"spent nearly three years"** James Mom, *President's Newsletter*, March 1983, p. 4.

page 162: **"one of the most significant accomplishments..."** "Report of the Board of Directors," *Radiologic Technology*, November/December 1983, p. 655.

page 163: **"The Secretary has failed..."** From an Aug. 13, 1985, letter to ASRT members, written by Roland Clements.

page 163: **"This situation reveals..."** Ralph Nader was quoted in an Oct. 10, 1985, *Washington Post* article titled "HHS Shields Itself from X-Ray Law."

page 163: **"further fragmentation..."** From "Committee Studying Restructure of the Society," *Radiologic Technology,* Vol. 51, No. 3, p. 363.

pages 165, 167-171: Information on the chronology of majority representation can be found in "ASRT Majority Representation Chronology," *ASRT Scanner,* April/May 1991, p. 7.

page 165: **"The time has come..."** Bill May, "Presidential Message," *Radiologic Technology*, May/June 1984, p. 184.

page 167: **"soliciting nominations..."** Phyllis Thompson, "ASRT Majority Representation Chronology," *ASRT Scanner*, April/May 1991, p. 7.

page 168: **"broadest spectrum..."** From "ASRT Majority Representation Chronology," *ASRT Scanner,* April/May 1991, p. 7.

page 168: **"the radiologists' maneuvers..."** From "ASRT Majority Representation Chronology," *ASRT Scanner*, April/May 1991, p. 7.

page 169: **"two additional technologists..."** From *ASRT House of Delegates Resolutions Adopted, Defeated and/or Withdrawn,* Section 1991, 91-108, p. 2.

page 169: Quotes from Bill May about majority representation are from "Majority Representation!" *RS Wavelength*, November 1991, p. 8.

page 169: **"This accomplishment would not have occurred..."** From "JRC Majority Representation!" *ASRT Scanner,* October/November 1991, p. 6.

page 171: Information on the Maryland Society sponsored resolution was found in "Resolutions Aplenty," ASRT Scanner, April/May 1990, p. 4; and in "Draft 5 Ok'd But Not Without Revisions," *RS Wavelength,* August/September 1990, p. 8.

page 172: **"No change at the ARRT..."** Jerry Reid, "Continuing Education Quiz," May/June 1994 *Radiologic Technology*, pp. 305-306.

page 172: **"Continuing education allows technologists..."** Jerry Reid, "CE Requirements for Certification Renewal," March/April 1994 *Radiologic Technology*, pp. 257-258.

page 173: **"I believe this mandate..."** Darrell McKay, "Forecast for the Next 100 Years," December 1993 *ASRT Scanner*, p. 2.

page 173: **"increasing professionalism in health professions..."** From "CAHEA Dissolves," *RS Wavelength*, December 1992, pp. 1-2.

page 173: **"not compromise the independence..."** From "Higher Education Act of 1992," *ACERT News*, March 1993, p. 2.

page 174: Information on JRCERT compliance with the Higher Education Act of 1992 can be found in "On the Path to Independence," *Radiologic Technology*, September/October 1994, pp. 61-62.

page 174: **"The requirements of the Higher Education Act..."** Marilyn Fay, "Why JRCERT Accreditation Is Worth It," *Radiologic Technology*, January/February 1995, pp. 193.

pages 174-175: Information comparing the JRCERT *Essentials* with the more generic *Standards* came from *Standards for an Accredited Education Program in Radiologic Sciences,* April 1995 Draft. JRCERT, Chicago, Ill.

page 175: Statistics on accredited radiography and radiation therapy programs came from *JRCERT Annual Report.* January 1995. JRCERT, Chicago, Ill.

page 175: Data from the ARRT survey is reported in "Demographics Are Us" by Jerry Reid, January/February 1991 *Radiologic Technology*, p. 234-236.

Illustration Credits

Unless otherwise noted, all illustrations credited to Charles C Thomas Publisher are from *The Trail of the Invisible Light* by E.R.N. Grigg, copyright 1965 by Charles C Thomas Publisher, Springfield, Ill; and all illustrations credited to Mosby Yearbook are from *Radiology: An Illustrated History* by Ronald Eisenberg, copyright 1992 by Mosby Yearbook, St. Louis, Mo.

Page

1   Roentgen woodcut: Charles C Thomas Publisher, Springfield, Ill.

3   Roentgen in lab: National Library of Medicine, Washington, D.C.

5   Static machine: National Library of Medicine, Washington, D.C. Wolfram Fuchs lab: Eastman Kodak Company, Rochester, N.Y. Anna Roentgen's hand: Otto Glasser, *Wilhelm Conrad Roentgen and the History of Roentgen Rays*, Charles C Thomas Publisher, Springfield, Ill., 1933

9   Portrait William Herbert Rollins: Charles C Thomas Publisher, Springfield, Ill.

10 Electrical Exposition: Burndy Library, Cambridge, Mass. Portrait Clarence Dally: Charles C Thomas Publisher, Springfield, Ill.

11 Portrait Heber Robarts: Mosby Year Book, St. Louis, Mo. Cover of *The American X-Ray Journal*: Mosby Year Book, St. Louis, Mo.

14 Charity Hospital X-Ray Department: Tulane University Department of Radiology, New Orleans, La.

15 Schiedel-Western fluoroscopic machine: Tulane University Department of Radiology, New Orleans La.

17 Kassabian's Roentgen-ray lab: Permission granted by Ronald L. Eisenberg. GE tube: Copyright General Electric. Reprinted courtesy General Electric Company, Milwaukee, Wis. First ARRS meeting: Mosby Year Book, St. Louis, Mo.

18 Portrait Russell D. Carman: Mayo Foundation, Rochester, Minn.

20 Early x-ray therapy session: Art Resource Inc., New York, N.Y.

23 World War I x-ray setup: National Atomic Museum, Albuquerque, N.M.

24 Portrait Marie Curie: National Atomic Museum, Albuquerque, N.M.

25 Marie Curie in lab: National Atomic Museum, Albuquerque, N.M.

27 Ed Jerman and static machine: Copyright General Electric. Reprinted courtesy General Electric Company, Milwaukee, Wis.

29 Electro-Therapeutic Manufacturing Co. Ad: Charles C Thomas Publisher, Springfield, Ill.

33 Ed Jerman's 1918 x-ray class: ASRT Archive, Albuquerque, N.M.

36 Electronic impulse x-ray timer: ASRT Archive, Albuquerque, N.M.

37 Radiology Became Exact ad: ASRT Archive, Albuquerque, N.M. Start Modernizing Now ad: ASRT Archive, Albuquerque, N.M.

39 Portrait ASRT founding members: ASRT Archive, Albuquerque, N.M. Portrait Ed C. Jerman: American Registry of Radiologic Technologists, St. Paul, Minn.

44 Portrait Edward Gunson: ASRT Archive, Albuquerque, N.M.

47 *The X-Ray Technician* cover: ASRT Archive, Albuquerque, N.M.

49 X-ray room at St. Francis Hospital: Archives of Sisters of the Third Order of St. Francis, Peoria, Ill.

51 Nun and child in x-ray room at St. Francis Hospital: Archives of Sisters of the Third Order of St. Francis, Peoria, Ill.

53 Nurse and patient: Art Resource Inc., New York, N.Y. Aurora x-ray table ad: ASRT Archive, Albuquerque, N.M. Mass chest x-rays: Reprinted with permission of the American Lung Association, New York, N.Y.

56 Portrait Alfred B. Greene: American Registry of Radiologic Technologists, St. Paul, Minn.

59 Portrait Jerman family: Personal collection of Virginia Milligan, Sun City, Ariz.

61 Pregnancy x-ray: ASRT Archive, Albuquerque, N.M.

63 Radiologic technology students at St. Louis University: ASRT Archive, Albuquerque, N.M.

64 Children line up for x-rays: Reprinted with permission of the American Lung Association, New York, N.Y.

65 Minnesota residents line-up for chest x-rays: Copyright General Electric. Reprinted courtesy of General Electric Company, Milwaukee, Wis.

67 Army School of Roentgen-ology assembling x-ray unit: U.S. Army Medical Department, Office of the Surgeon General, Washington, D.C. Picker adver-tisement: ASRT Archive, Albuquerque, N.M.

68 Seminar in diagnostic radi-ology: U.S. Army Medical Department, Office of Sur-geon General, Washington, D.C.

69 Class of Army Roentgeno-logy Students: U.S. Army Medical Department, Office of Surgeon General, Washington, D.C. .

71 Radiographer-in-training: ASRT Archive, Albuquerque, N.M.

72 Mobile x-ray unit: U.S. Army Medical Department, Office of the Surgeon General, Washington, D.C.

74 Wounded serviceman: U.S. Army Medical Department, Office of the Surgeon General, Washington, D.C.

75 Army radiographer using shell casing: ASRT Archive, Albuquerque, N.M.

76 Portrait of Arthur Fuchs: ASRT Archive, Albuquerque, N.M.

78 Portrait of Rose Marie Pegues-Perkins: Courtesy of the family of Rose Marie Pegues-Perkins and Alan Oestreich, M.D., Child-ren's Hospital Medical Center, Cincinnati, Ohio.

79 Portrait of Ted Ott: Personal collection of Theodore T. Ott, Los Angeles, Calif.

81 Radiation safety: ASRT Archive, Albuquerque, N.M. Reed x-ray technic computer: ASRT Archives, Albuquerque, N.M.

83 Civil defense program: ASRT Archive, Albuquerque, N.M.

86 Class of 1952, Johns Hopkins University: ASRT Archive, Albuquerque, N.M. Portrait of Richard Olden: ASRT Archive, Albuquerque, N.M.

89 Portrait of Genevieve Eilert: ASRT Archives, Albuquerque, N.M.

90 Genevieve Eilert at Fond du Lac office: Personal collection of Genevieve J. Eilert, Fond du Lac, Wis.

92 Annual Conference: Personal collection of Jack and Angie Cullinan, Rochester, N.Y.

95 Jack Cullinan lecture: Personal collection of Jack and Angie Cullinan, Rochester, N.Y. John Cahoon and students: Duke University Archives, Durham, N.C.

96 Portrait of Sr. Mary Alacoque Anger: ASRT Archive, Albuquerque, N.M.

97 Portrait of Royce Osborn: ASRT Archive, Albuquerque, N.M.

98 Royce Osborn: Personal collection of Royce Osborn, Carson, Calif.

100 John Cahoon as a student: Duke University Archives, Durham, N.C.

101 Portrait of John B. Cahoon: ASRT Archive, Albuquerque, N.M.

102 Portrait of Bill Conklin: Personal collection of Bill Conklin, Orangeburg, S.C.

103 Portrait of Margaret Hoing: ASRT Archive, Albuquerque, N.M.

104 Portrait of Virginia Milligan: ASRT Archive, Albuquerque, N.M. Portrait of Ruth Jaffke: ASRT Archive, Albuquerque, N.M.

105 Portrait of Jean Widger: ASRT Archive, Albuquerque, N.M.

106 –

108 Photos of Jack and Angie Cullinan: Personal collec-tion of Jack and Angie Cullinan, Rochester, N.Y.

111 Examining wounded sol-dier: Personal collection of Juris Patrylak, New Haven, Conn. Westinghouse ad: ASRT Archive, Albuquer-que, N.M.

112 Office in Chicago: ASRT Archive, Albuquerque, N.M.

113 ASRT Officers: ASRT Archive, Albuquerque, N.M.

114 –

115 Vietnam photos: Personal collection of Juris Patrylak, New Haven, Conn.

118 Photo of Ward Keller, Sen. Randolph and Sr. Agnes Therese: Personal collec-tion of Ward Keller, Placitas, N.M.

120 First battery-powered mobile x-ray unit: ASRT Archive, Albuquerque, N.M.

121 Letter from Patricia Nixon: ASRT Archive, Albuquer-que, N.M.

122 Portrait of Ward Keller: ASRT Archive, Albuquer-que, N.M.

125 Department chief with Caroline Strong Steele: ASRT Archive, Albuquer-que, N.M.

126 Caroline Strong Steele: ASRT Archive, Albuquer-que, N.M.

129 William Coolidge: ASRT Archive, Albuquerque, N.M. Measurement of young girl's tyroid function: HP Publishers, New York, N.Y.

131 Therapy unit at Mercy Hospital: Reprinted courtesy of General Electric Company, Milwaukee, Wis.

132 Picker shock-proof therapy unit: Courtesy Picker International, Cleveland, Ohio. Million-volt x-ray therapy unit: U.S. Army Medical Department, Office of the Surgeon General, Washington, D.C.

134 Mock-up of Cobalt 60 unit: ASRT Archive, Albuquerque, N.M.

135 Portrait of Varian brothers: Varian Associates, Palo Alto, Calif.

136 Portrait Eileen McCullough: ASRT Archive, Albuquerque, N.M.

138 Portrait of Phyllis Thompson: ASRT Archive, Albuquerque, N.M.

139 Portrait of Beverly Buck: ASRT Archive, Albuquerque, N.M.

140 Portrait of Carole Sullivan: Personal collection of Carole Sullivan, Oklahoma City, Okla.

141 Cover of *Radiation Therapist*: ASRT Archive, Albuquerque, N.M.

142 Stereotactic radiotherapy: Varian Associates, Palo Alto, Calif.

145 Computed tomography: General Electric Medical Systems, Waukesha, Wis.

146 Portrait of LaVerne Gurley: Personal collection of LaVerne Gurley, Memphis, Tenn.

149 Ultrasound: Courtesy Philips Medical Systems, Shelton, Conn.

151 Nuclear medicine: Mallinckrodt Medical Inc., St. Louis, Mo.

152 Magnetic resonance imaging: Siemens Medical Systems, Iselin, N.J.

155 ISRRT Conference: ASRT Archive, Albuquerque, N.M. Triad meeting: ASRT Archive, Albuquerque, N.M.

156 Portrait of Ward Keller: ASRT Archive, Albuquerque, N.M.

158 Portrait of James A. Mom: ASRT Archive, Albuquerque, N.M.

159 Portrait of Marilyn Lloyd: Personal collection of Marilyn Lloyd, Washington, D.C.

161 American Cancer Society mammography conference: Courtesy the American Cancer Society, New York, N.Y.

162 ASRT offices, past and present: ASRT Archive, Albuquerque, N.M.

164 House of Delegates drawing: ASRT Archive, Albuquerque, N.M.

165 Portrait of Joan Parsons: ASRT Archive, Albuquerque, N.M.

168 Portraits of Bill May, Linda Wingfield and Roland Clements: ASRT Archive, Albuquerque, N.M.

169 Portrait of Becky Kruse: ASRT Archive, Albuquerque, N.M.

170 –

171 ARRT majority representation: ASRT Archive, Albuquerque, N.M.

172 Portrait of Jerry Reid: American Registry of Radiologic Technologists, St. Paul, Minn.

175 Portrait of Marilyn Fay: ASRT Archive, Albuquerque, N.M.

176 ASRT Educational Consensus Conference: ASRT Archive, Albuquerque, N.M.

179 –

192 All photos: ASRT Archive, Albuquerque, N.M.

DATE DUE

JUN 20 '96			
JUL 1 0 '96			
SEP 1 0 97			
GAYLORD			PRINTED IN U.S.A.